QUICK *&* EASY DINNERS

100 Quick and Easy Dinners from Around the World — Ready in Under 15 Minutes

By: Indigo Chen

Copyright 2025
All rights reserved.

All rights reserved. No part of this book may be reproduced, stored in a retrieval system, or transmitted in any form or by any means, mechanical or electronic, including photocopying or recording, without written permission from the author. Brief passages may be quoted in reviews with proper attribution.

Disclaimer
Despite every attempt to ensure the accuracy of the information in this publication, neither the author nor the publisher takes responsibility for any errors, omissions, or differing interpretations of the subject matter contained herein.

This book is intended for entertainment and informational purposes only. The views expressed are those of the author and should not be taken as professional or expert advice. The reader is responsible for their own actions and decisions. Compliance with all applicable laws and regulations, including those related to professional licensing, business practices, and advertising, is the sole responsibility of the reader. This includes adhering to international, federal, state, and local laws applicable to conducting business or personal activities in any jurisdiction.

Neither the author nor the publisher assumes any responsibility or liability whatsoever on behalf of any purchaser or reader of these materials. Any perceived slight of any individual or organization is entirely unintentional.

Please note that similarities with already published recipes are possible.

TABLE OF CONTENTS

TABLE OF CONTENTS 3
INTRODUCTION 4
GETTING STARTED 11

    Why Fast Doesn't Mean Flavorless 12

    Must-Have Pantry Staples 13

    Must-Have Tools & Equipment 15

    Prep Like a Pro 16

    Quick Dinner Tips and Tricks 17

JAPANESE DINNERS 18

    1. Sesame-Crusted Salmon 19

    2. Sweet Miso Steak with Ramen 21

    3. Chicken Teriyaki Donburi Bowl 23

    4. Zaru Soba (Chilled Soba Noodles) 25

    5. Gyudon (Japanese Beef Rice Bowl) 27

    6. Tamagoyaki with Rice 29

    7. Miso Glazed Cod 31

    8. Japanese Curry Udon 33

MEDITERRANEAN DINNERS 35

    9. Pasta with Spinach and Walnut Pesto 36

    10. Herb Shrimp Pasta 38

    11. Pesto Zucchini Noodles with Grilled Chicken 40

12. Chicken Souvlaki with Tzatziki 42
13. Tuna and White Bean Salad 44
14. Grilled Eggplant and Halloumi Stacks 46
15. Garlic Shrimp with Lemon Couscous 48
16. Lemon Pasta with Spinach and Feta 50
17. Chickpea and Olive Skillet with Harissa 52
18. Herb-Crusrted Lamb Chops 54

AMERICAN DINNERS 56

19. Almond-Crusted Salmon with Salad 57
20. Lemon Herb Grilled Chicken 59
21. Seared Scallops with Spinach 61
22. Cod with Sautéed Spinach 63
23. Sweet Potato Noodles with Spinach 65
24. Steak Bites with Garlic Butter 67
25. BBQ Chicken Wraps 69
26. Classic Patty Melt 71
27. Cheesy Chicken Quesadillas 73
28. Chili Cheese Dogs 75

MEXICAN DINNERS 77

29. Fish Tacos with Pico de Gallo 78
30. Chipotle Shrimp Tacos 80

31. Beef and Black Bean Quesadilla 82
32. Chicken Fajita Skillet 84
33. Carne Asada Street Tacos 86
34. Chorizo and Potato Skillet 88
35. Chicken Tinga Tostadas 90
36. Veggie Fajita Tacos 92
37. Beef Picadillo Tacos 94
38. Sopa de Lima (Yucatán Lime Soup) 96

ITALIAN DINNERS 98

39. Creamy Pesto Gnocchi 99
40. Caprese Chicken Cutlets 101
41. Garlic Butter Shrimp Spaghetti 103
42. Italian Sausage and Pepper Skillet 105
43. Spinach and Ricotta Stuffed Portobellos 107
44. Prosciutto and Arugula Flatbread 109
45. Pasta Aglio e Olio 111
46. Chicken Piccata 113
47. Margherita Skillet Pizza 115
48. Tuna Puttanesca 117
49. Chicken Marsala Skillet 119
50. White Bean and Kale Sauté 121

INDIAN DINNERS ....
123
- 51. Egg Curry (Anda Curry) ....
  124
- 52. Jeera Rice with Tadka Dal ....
  126
- 53. Spinach and Paneer Curry ....
  128
- 54. Quick Chicken Korma ....
  130
- 55. Achari Chicken (Pickled-Spiced Chicken) ....
  132
- 56. Mixed Vegetable Curry ....
  134
- 57. Chicken Jalfrezi ....
  136
- 58. Baked Tandoori Chicken Curry ....
  138
- 59. Easy Mutton Karahi ....
  140
- 60. Indian Fish Curry ....
  142

THAI DINNERS ....
144
- 61. Pad Kra Pao (Thai Basil Chicken) ....
  145
- 62. Thai Shrimp Red Curry ....
  147
- 63. Thai Glass Noodle Stir-Fry (Pad Woon Sen) ....
  149
- 64. Thai Chicken Lettuce Wraps ....
  151
- 65. Tom Yum Soup (Thai Hot and Sour Soup) ....
  153

MIDDLE EASTERN DINNERS ....
155
- 66. Chicken Shawarma Wrap Bowls ....
  156
- 67. Spiced Lamb and Eggplant Skillet ....
  158
- 68. Za'atar Chicken with Hummus and Pita ....
  160

69. Chickpea and Spinach Stew 162
70. Kofta Rice Bowl with Tahini 164
71. Ful Medames with Fried Egg and Pita 166

EUROPEAN DINNERS 168

72. Scandinavian Salmon with Dill Yogurt Sauce 169
73. German Pork Schnitzel with Lemon and Greens 171
74. Quick Hungarian Goulash 173
75. French Ratatouille Stir-Fry 175

VIETNAMESE DINNERS 177

76. Vietnamese Shaking Beef 178
77. Vietnamese Lemongrass Chicken 180
78. Vietnamese Skillet Egg Meatloaf 182
79. Beef and Water Spinach Stir-Fry 184
80. Vietnamese Tamarind Shrimp 186

CHINESE DINNERS 188

81. Chicken Manchurian 189
82. Beef and Mushroom Noodles with Broth 191
83. Beef and Broccoli Stir-Fry 193
84. Chinese Tomato and Egg Stir-Fry 195
85. Kung Pao Chicken 197
86. Chinese Pepper Steak 199

- 87. Garlic Bok Choy with Tofu 201
- 88. Tofu and Mushroom Stir-Fry 203
- 89. Ginger Sesame Chicken Stir-Fry 205
- 90. Salmon Fried Rice 207

MALAYSIAN DINNERS 209

- 91. Ayam Kicap (Soy Sauce Chicken Stir-Fry) 210
- 92. Sambal Prawns (Udang Masak Sambal) 212
- 93. Mee Goreng Mamak (Spicy Fried Noodles) 214
- 94. Sardine Curry 216
- 95. Ikan Bakar (Pan-Grilled Fish) 218
- 96. Malaysian Chicken Kurma 220

KOREAN DINNERS 222

- 97. Bulgogi Beef Skillet 223
- 98. Kimchi Fried Rice (Kimchi Bokkeumbap) 225
- 99. Gochujang Chicken Stir-Fry 227
- 100. Korean Tofu Stew (Sundubu Jjigae) 229

CONCLUSION 231

INTRODUCTION

Dinner — that final, grounding meal that marks the close of a long day. Across the globe, dinner brings families together, nourishes bodies, and tells the stories of generations through spices, staples, and the rhythm of the stove. But in the chaos of modern life, the idea of a home-cooked dinner can feel daunting, even impossible. That's exactly why this cookbook exists.

Quick & Easy Dinner Cookbook is your passport to fast, flavorful meals that don't compromise on quality, culture, or nourishment. Every recipe in this collection is designed to be made from start to finish in 15 minutes or less — no slow braising, no complex prep, no fancy appliances required. Just simple, satisfying meals from the world's dinner tables, streamlined for busy lives.

Whether you're a student cooking in a tiny kitchen, a parent juggling work and after-school chaos, or a beginner learning how to pan-fry without fear, this book is for you. We've sourced, tested, and trimmed recipes inspired by the cuisines of over 30 countries — from Vietnamese Lemongrass Chicken and Moroccan Chickpea Skillet to Tex-Mex BBQ Wraps and comforting Indian Curries — ensuring that every dish respects its roots while fitting your real-life time limits.

But this isn't just a shortcut collection. It's also a celebration of global traditions, a crash course in efficient kitchen habits, and a reminder that a delicious, nourishing meal doesn't have to take hours. You'll find pantry-smart tips, clever prep shortcuts, and an entire section on essential tools and time-saving techniques to help you cook smarter, not harder.

This book is not just about eating quickly — it's about cooking confidently, exploring flavors beyond your routine, and creating moments of joy at the dinner table even on your busiest days. From vegetarian to meaty, one-pan to no-cook, you'll discover recipes that suit every palate and lifestyle.

So roll up your sleeves, grab a skillet or a spoon, and get ready to change the way you think about fast food — because with the right recipe, a global dinner can happen in less time than it takes to wait for delivery.

GETTING STARTED

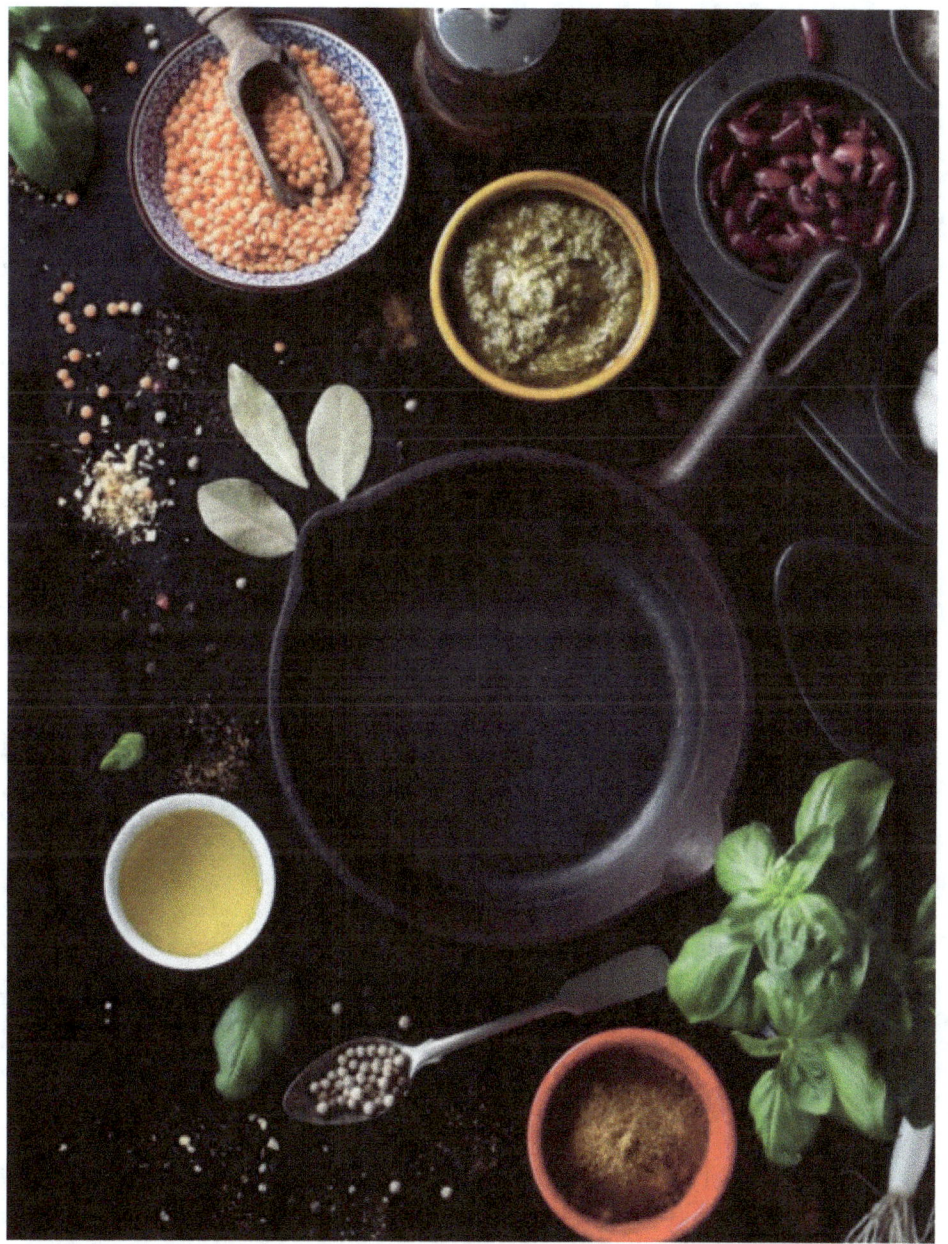

Why Fast Doesn't Mean Flavorless

There's a common misconception in cooking: that a delicious dish must simmer for hours or require a long list of ingredients. Yet, across cultures and cuisines, countless quick meals prove that speed in the kitchen can still yield vibrant, satisfying flavors. Here's why fast cooking doesn't mean sacrificing taste:

Flavor Comes from Technique, Not Time
Mastering quick techniques—like searing, sautéing, toasting spices, or finishing with a bright splash of lemon or vinegar—builds deep, complex flavors without hours of cooking. It's not about slow-cooking; it's about cooking smart.

Global Cuisines Perfect Speed and Flavor
From Japan's gyudon beef bowls to Mexico's zesty tacos, many traditional dishes are crafted to be prepared quickly yet bursting with personality. These recipes often lean on bold seasonings, fresh ingredients, and aromatic herbs rather than prolonged cooking.

Bold Ingredients = Instant Flavor Boost
Flavor powerhouses such as garlic, ginger, chilies, soy sauce, mustard, and vinegars elevate dishes in seconds. A drizzle of toasted sesame oil or a pinch of smoked paprika can instantly transform a simple meal.

Prep Ahead to Maximize Flavor and Efficiency
Organizing your mise en place—having sauces, spice blends, and chopped aromatics ready—means you can assemble flavorful meals in no time. Even a quick stir-fry becomes remarkable with thoughtful preparation.

Smart Shortcuts Enhance, Not Diminish
Using quality store-bought curry pastes, rotisserie chicken, or pre-cut veggies isn't taking shortcuts on flavor—it's working smarter. These helpers drastically reduce cooking time while preserving, or sometimes even enhancing, taste.

Quick Meals Can Be Fully Balanced
Speedy dishes still hit the essential flavor profiles—savory, sweet, acidic, and spicy—by thoughtfully combining ingredients. It's how flavors work together, not how long they cook, that creates a satisfying meal.

Must-Have Pantry Staples

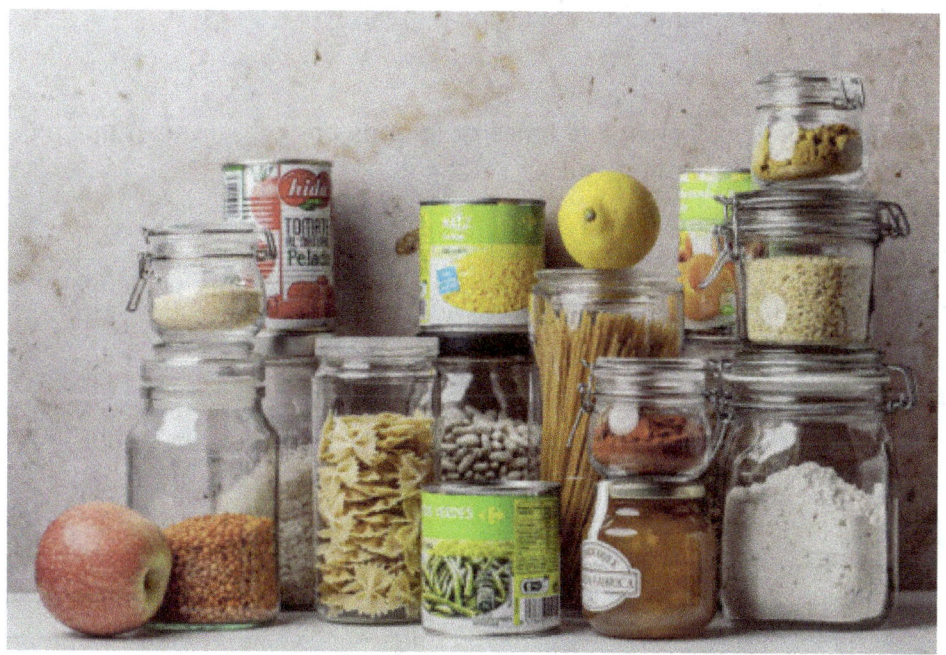

Building a well-stocked pantry is the first step to becoming a confident and creative cook. These essential ingredients form the base of countless fast dinners — ready in minutes without ever turning on the oven.

Salt & Pepper
The backbone of all seasoning. Store salt in an airtight container with a small spoon to prevent clumping and for easy measuring. Use freshly ground pepper for best flavor.

Sugar
White sugar for sauces or quick dressings. Brown sugar can add depth to marinades and glazes.

Oil
Olive oil for finishing or dressings, and a neutral oil (like canola or vegetable) for sautéing and frying.

Butter (Optional)
Table butter adds richness to sauces and skillet dishes. Store in the fridge and use sparingly to build flavor fast.

Spices & Dried Herbs

Start with essentials like chili flakes, cumin, paprika, black pepper, turmeric, oregano, thyme, and garlic powder. These can transform the simplest ingredients into bold, global meals.

Aromatics
Garlic, ginger, onions, and limes or lemons bring brightness, umami, and complexity to even the quickest dishes.

Flour (Minimal Use)
Keep a small amount for thickening sauces or coating proteins for pan-frying. Skip any baking-specific flours.

Broths & Stocks
Store cartons or bouillon cubes of chicken, beef, or vegetable broth to enrich soups, stews, and skillet sauces quickly.

Canned & Jarred Goods
Chickpeas, beans, crushed tomatoes, tuna, olives, coconut milk, pesto, curry pastes, and harissa — all high-impact, low-effort additions.

Grains & Noodles
Instant rice, couscous, soba noodles, or ramen — perfect for one-pan or microwave cooking.

Frozen Vegetables
Keep frozen corn, spinach, peas, and mixed veggies for effortless stir-fries, curries, and soups.

Protein Staples
Canned tuna, cooked rotisserie chicken (shredded and frozen), frozen shrimp, and quick-cook tofu or paneer can be ready in minutes.

Must-Have Tools & Equipment

You don't need a fancy kitchen or expensive gadgets to cook great food — just the right tools for the job. Whether you're living in a small apartment, starting out on your own, or just short on time, these essential items help you prep, cook, and clean up faster. Think of them as your kitchen sidekicks: reliable, straightforward, and ready to work with your microwave, stovetop, or skillet. No ovens. No mixers. No stress.

Cookware
- 4-Quart Saucepan – Ideal for boiling rice, pasta, noodles, or soup.
- Non-stick Skillets (8" & 12") – Essential for stir-frying, sautéing, and one-pan meals.
- Metal Skillet – For getting that perfect sear on meat or veggies.
- Cutting Board & Knives – Paring and chef's knives cover most slicing, chopping, and dicing.
- Colander – Drains pasta, canned beans, and veggies fast.
- Tongs, Wooden Spoons & Spatulas – For flipping, stirring, and tossing ingredients with ease.
- Prep Bowls & Mixing Bowls – For prepping, marinating, or assembling meals.

Everyday Tools
- Measuring Cups & Spoons – Accuracy helps with fast, consistent meals.
- Box Grater & Vegetable Peeler – For shredding cheese or peeling carrots/potatoes.
- Citrus Juicer or Reamer – Quick flavor boost from lemons or limes.
- Whisk – Great for vinaigrettes or scrambled eggs.
- Can Opener – Since pantry meals often involve canned goods.
- Instant-Read Thermometer – Ensures proteins are safely cooked without guesswork.

Appliances
- Microwave – Reheats leftovers, steams veggies, and cooks rice in a pinch.
- Stovetop Burner (Gas or Induction) – Core of all quick cooking.
- Blender – For sauces, soups, or smoothies.
- Toaster – Useful for reheating or toasting bread, pita, or wraps.
- Electric Kettle – Boils water quickly for couscous, ramen, or broth-based dishes.
- Mini Food Processor (Optional) – Speeds up chopping and blending.

Prep Like a Pro

Great meals don't start with fancy ingredients or expensive equipment — they start with smart prep. Whether you're cooking for one or feeding a crowd, getting organized before you turn on the stove makes dinner faster, smoother, and way less stressful.

Here's how to prep like a pro — even if you're just getting started:

Read the Recipe First
Always take a minute to read the full recipe before you begin. This helps you understand what comes first, what needs time (like marinating or simmering), and what you can prep ahead. Surprises belong in birthday parties, not in dinner.

Set Up Your Station (a.k.a. Mise en Place)
The French call it mise en place — everything in its place. That means measuring out spices, chopping veggies, draining cans, and having all your ingredients within reach before you start cooking. It may feel like extra work, but it saves time (and panic) later.

Keep a Trash Bowl Nearby
This simple tip can be a game changer. Instead of running back and forth to the trash, use a mixing bowl or container to collect scraps while you prep. When you're done, dump it once. Clean counter, clean workflow.

Use Time-Savers
Don't shy away from shortcuts. Pre-chopped veggies, canned beans, frozen garlic cubes, rotisserie chicken — they're all fair game in a busy kitchen. What matters is that dinner gets made and you enjoy the process.

Clean as You Go
Wipe down your board, rinse your knife, toss empty cans. Tidying as you cook helps avoid overwhelm and makes cleanup a breeze after dinner's done. It's the secret behind every confident home cook.

Store Smart
Use zip bags, clear containers, or jars to keep chopped produce, sauces, or pre-measured ingredients ready for the next day. Label and date them if needed — your future self will thank you.

Quick Dinner Tips and Tricks

Dinner in 15 minutes? Yes, it's totally possible — with the right habits and a few clever shortcuts. Whether you're cooking after a long day or just don't want to spend hours in the kitchen, these quick tips will help you pull it off with ease.

Plan Just One Step Ahead
You don't need a full weekly meal plan. But knowing what's for dinner tonight means you can defrost meat, pre-cook grains, or grab ingredients earlier — saving time when the hunger hits.

Use One-Pan Meals
Skillets, stir-fries, and sheet pan dinners are your best friends. Less cookware means less cleanup, and cooking everything together builds flavor fast. Look for recipes that combine protein, veggies, and sauce in one go.

Pre-Cut Veggies = Time Saved
Buy pre-cut onions, sliced mushrooms, coleslaw mix, or chopped bell peppers. They cut prep time drastically, and they're worth it on busy days. Or, prep your own in batches and store them in airtight containers.

Double Up, Freeze Down
Making rice? Cook double. Saucing ground beef? Make extra and freeze half. A small effort now means a meal-ready shortcut later. Keep a few freezer-friendly staples for "emergency dinners."

Cans and Jars Are Heroes
Canned beans, tomatoes, coconut milk, sauces, broths — these pantry MVPs make dinner fast and flavorful. Rinse canned beans before using to reduce sodium and boost freshness.

Rotisserie Chicken: The Lifesaver
Shred it for wraps, toss it into stir-fries, or layer it into rice bowls. A cooked rotisserie chicken cuts out 30+ minutes and gives you at least two meals.

Don't Skip the Acid
A squeeze of lemon or splash of vinegar at the end of cooking can brighten flavors instantly. It's a quick trick that makes even simple meals taste fresh and balanced.

JAPANESE DINNERS

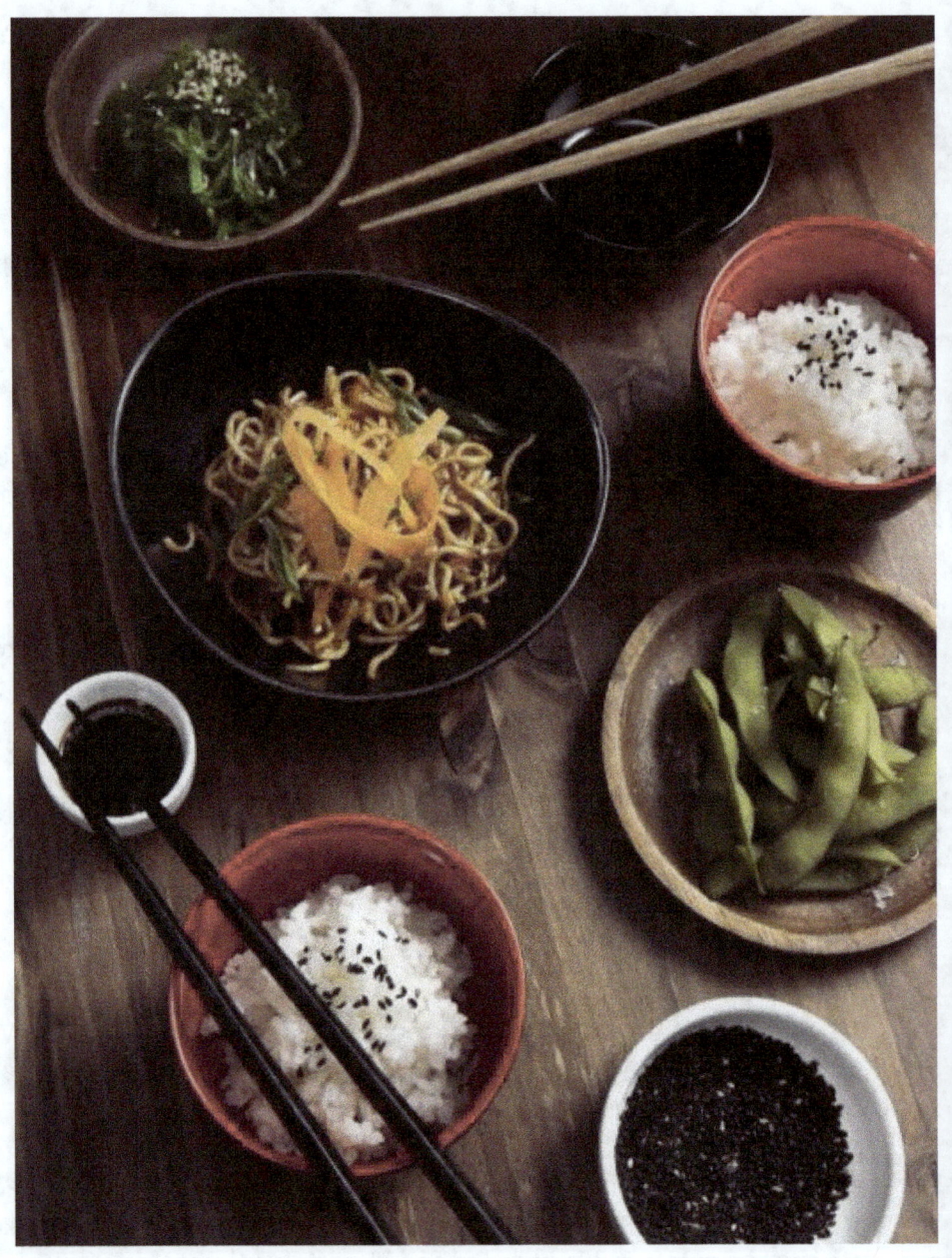

1. Sesame-Crusted Salmon

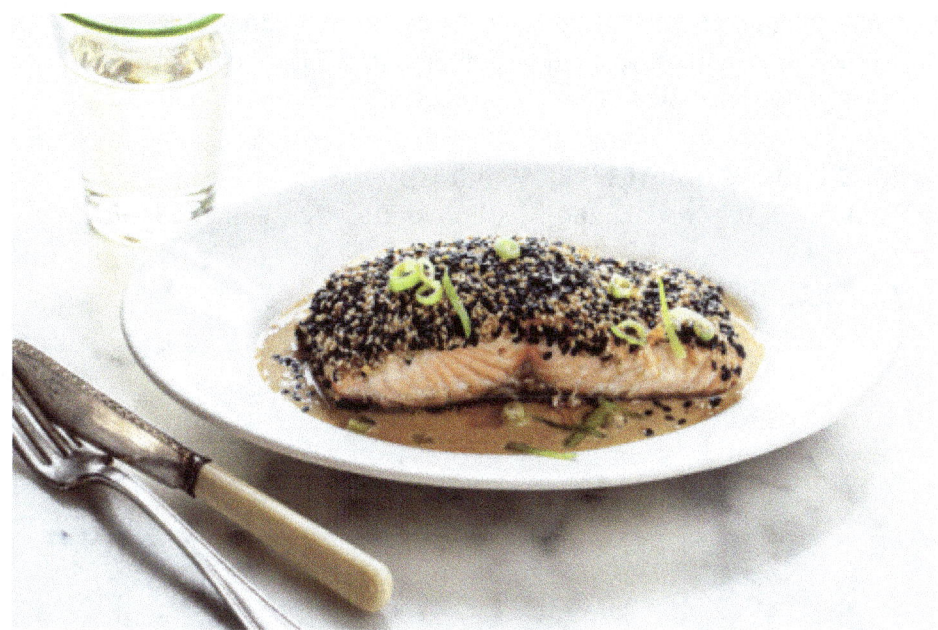

Prep Time: 10 minutes | Cook Time: 8 minutes | Makes: 4 servings

Sesame has been used in Japanese cuisine for centuries, especially in dishes like goma-ae (sesame-dressed vegetables) and as a garnish for rice and noodles. This sesame-crusted salmon blends traditional Japanese flavors with a modern twist. The crisp coating and soy-ginger sauce create a simple yet elegant meal that's deeply rooted in the country's appreciation for minimal, balanced flavors.

INGREDIENTS:
- 4 salmon fillets (about 6 oz each)
- 2 tablespoons sesame seeds
- 1 tablespoon olive oil
- Salt and pepper, to taste
- 1 tablespoon lemon juice
- 2 tablespoons soy sauce or tamari
- 1 teaspoon fresh ginger, grated
- 1 garlic clove, minced
- 1 tablespoon fresh parsley, chopped (optional, for garnish)

INSTRUCTIONS:
1. Season salmon with salt and pepper. Press sesame seeds on top to coat.

2. Heat oil in a skillet. Place salmon sesame-side down. Cook 3–4 minutes until golden.
3. Flip and cook other side for 3–4 minutes until done.
4. Mix lemon juice, soy sauce, ginger, and garlic in a bowl.
5. Drizzle sauce over salmon. Garnish with parsley if using.

NUTRITION ESTIMATES (PER SERVING):
Calories: 320 | Protein: 28g | Carbohydrates: 2g | Fat: 22g | Fiber: 0g

QUICK & EASY TIP:
Use boneless fillets and pre-grated ginger to cut down prep time.

2. Sweet Miso Steak with Ramen

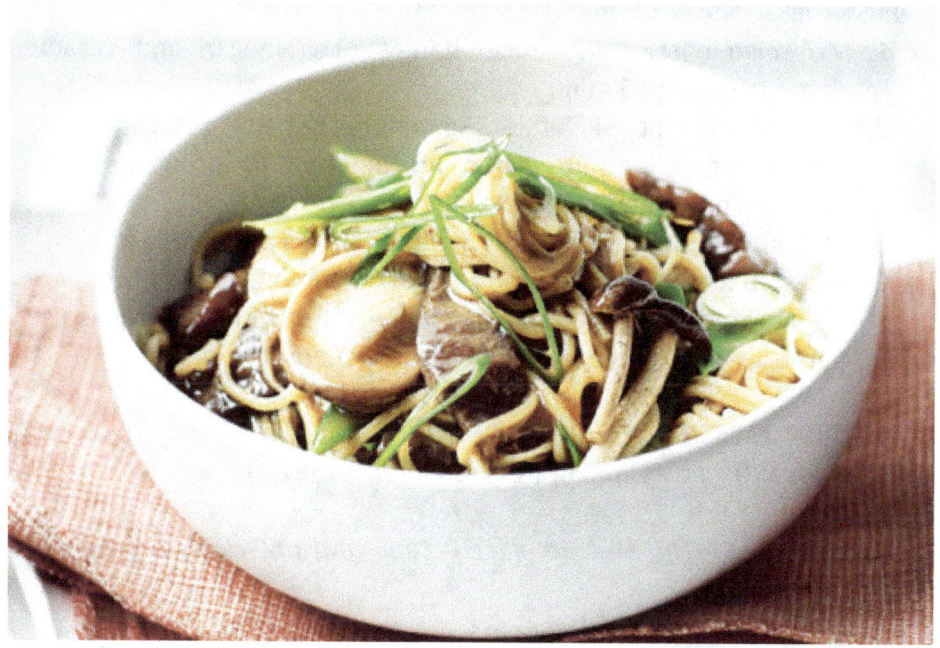

Prep Time: 20 minutes | Cook Time: 15 minutes | Makes: 4 servings

Miso, a fermented soybean paste, is a cornerstone of Japanese cooking known for its umami depth. In this comforting fusion bowl, sweet miso enhances marinated steak slices, served over tender ramen noodles in a savory broth with crisp vegetables. It's a modern twist on classic miso flavors and hearty ramen, perfect for cozy nights.

INGREDIENTS:
- 1 lb (450 g) flank steak, thinly sliced
- 2 tablespoons sweet miso paste
- 2 tablespoons soy sauce
- 2 tablespoons honey or maple syrup
- 2 tablespoons rice vinegar
- 1 tablespoon sesame oil
- 2 cloves garlic, minced
- 1 tablespoon fresh ginger, minced
- 4 cups beef broth
- 4 oz (115 g) ramen noodles
- 1 cup baby spinach
- 1 cup sliced mushrooms
- 1 cup shredded carrots
- 2 green onions, sliced

- 1 tablespoon sesame seeds (optional)

INSTRUCTIONS:
1. Mix miso paste, soy sauce, honey, rice vinegar, and sesame oil. Marinate steak for 15 minutes.
2. Sear steak in a hot skillet for 3–4 minutes per side. Set aside.
3. In the same skillet, sauté garlic and ginger for 30 seconds.
4. Add beef broth and bring to a simmer.
5. Add ramen noodles. Cook for 3 minutes or as per package.
6. Add spinach, mushrooms, and carrots. Simmer for 2 minutes.
7. Divide ramen and vegetables into bowls. Top with steak slices.
8. Garnish with green onions and sesame seeds if using.

NUTRITION ESTIMATES (PER SERVING):
Calories: 380 | Protein: 25g | Carbs: 40g | Fat: 12g | Fiber: 3g

QUICK & EASY TIP: Use pre-sliced steak and pre-washed greens to cut down prep time.

| 3. | Chicken Teriyaki Donburi Bowl |

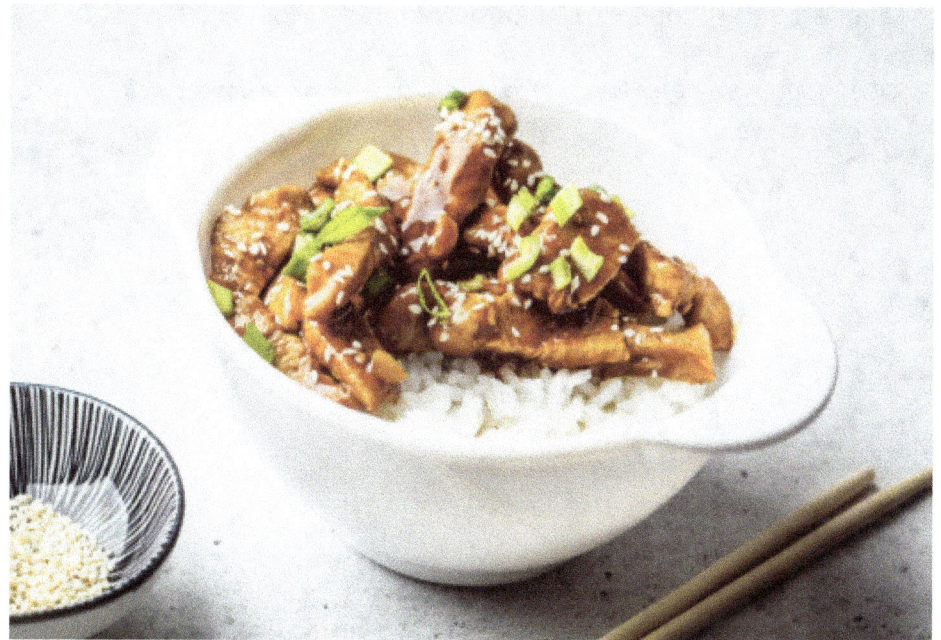

Prep Time: 5 minutes | Cook Time: 9 minutes | Makes: 2

Teriyaki is one of Japan's most famous cooking techniques, involving a glossy soy-based glaze. In this donburi (rice bowl) version, tender chicken is coated in a sweet-savory sauce and served over steamed rice for a balanced, comforting meal.

INGREDIENTS:
- 200g boneless chicken thighs, sliced
- 2 tbsp soy sauce
- 1 tbsp mirin
- 1 tbsp sugar
- 1 tsp sesame oil
- 1 tsp grated ginger
- 1 cup cooked Japanese rice
- Chopped green onions and sesame seeds, for garnish

INSTRUCTIONS:
1. Mix soy sauce, mirin, sugar, sesame oil, and ginger to make teriyaki sauce.
2. Sear chicken in a non-stick pan for 5–6 minutes until golden.
3. Pour sauce over chicken. Cook 2–3 minutes until thickened.
4. Serve over warm rice. Garnish with green onions and sesame seeds.

NUTRITION ESTIMATES (PER SERVING):
Calories: 520 | Protein: 31g | Carbs: 46g | Fat: 22g | Fiber: 1g

QUICK & EASY TIP: *Use microwave rice and pre-sliced chicken to speed up prep time.*

4. Zaru Soba (Chilled Soba Noodles)

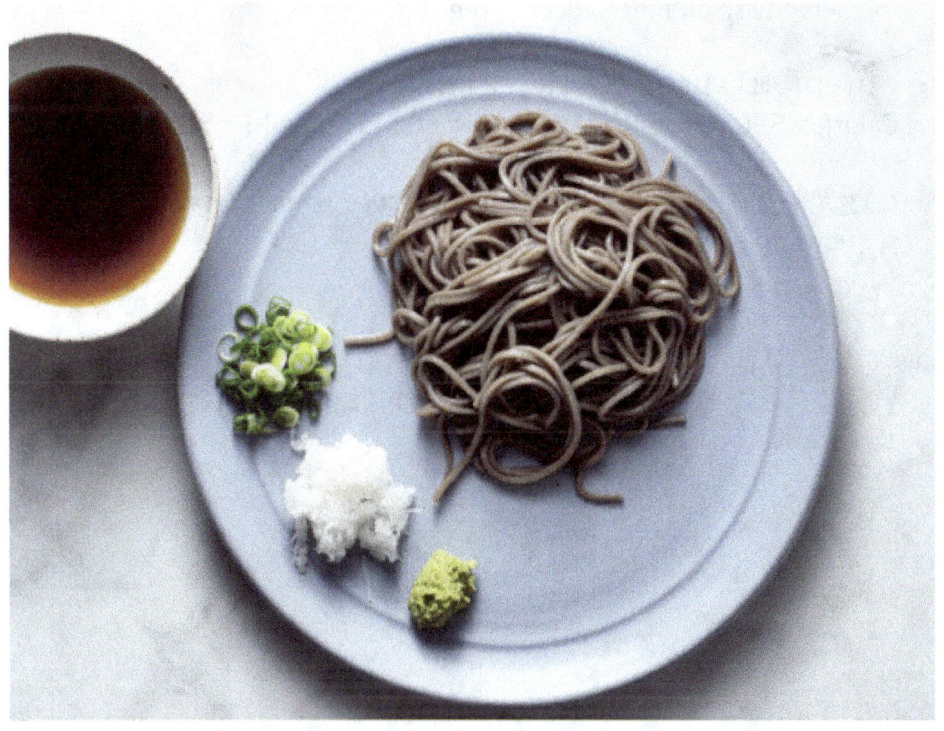

Prep Time: 3 minutes | Cook Time: 10 minutes | Makes: 2

Zaru soba is a beloved summer dinner in Japan, featuring cold buckwheat noodles served with a flavorful soy-based dipping sauce. It's light, refreshing, and requires minimal cooking — perfect for quick evenings or warm-weather meals.

INGREDIENTS:
- 160g dried soba noodles
- 2 tbsp soy sauce
- 2 tbsp mirin
- 2 tbsp dashi or water
- 1 tsp sugar
- Chopped green onions and shredded nori, to serve

INSTRUCTIONS:
1. Cook soba noodles according to package (usually 5–6 minutes). Rinse under cold water.
2. In a small bowl, mix soy sauce, mirin, dashi (or water), and sugar for the dipping sauce.

3. Plate noodles on a bamboo mat or dish. Garnish with green onions and nori.
4. Serve with dipping sauce on the side.

NUTRITION ESTIMATES (PER SERVING):
Calories: 390 | Protein: 13g | Carbs: 60g | Fat: 4g | Fiber: 2g

QUICK & EASY TIP: Prep the dipping sauce while the noodles cook — it requires no simmering.

5. Gyudon (Japanese Beef Rice Bowl)

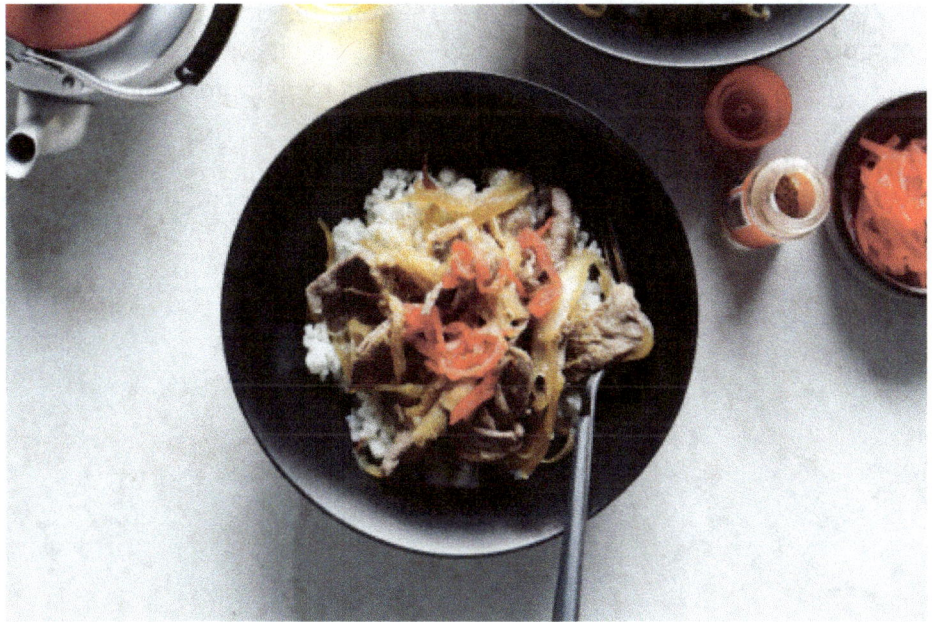

Prep Time: 4 minutes | Cook Time: 10 minutes | Makes: 2

Gyudon, meaning "beef bowl," is a beloved staple of Japanese comfort food. It became popular during the Meiji era (late 19th to early 20th century), when Western influences led to the introduction of beef into the Japanese diet. Served in casual eateries and home kitchens alike, Gyudon embodies the Japanese approach to fast food: nourishing, balanced, and deeply flavorful. It's the kind of dish you'll find at train stations, convenience chains like Yoshinoya, and even bento boxes—warm, quick, and satisfying.

INGREDIENTS:
- 200g thinly sliced beef (ribeye or sukiyaki cuts)
- ¼ onion, thinly sliced
- 2 tbsp soy sauce
- 1 tbsp mirin
- 1 tbsp sake (or water)
- 1 tsp sugar
- 1 tsp grated ginger (optional)
- 1 cup cooked Japanese rice
- Pickled ginger and scallions, for garnish

INSTRUCTIONS:

1. In a skillet, combine soy sauce, mirin, sake, sugar, and onion. Simmer 2 minutes.
2. Add beef and ginger. Cook for 5–6 minutes until beef is tender and sauce slightly thickens.
3. Serve over hot rice. Garnish with pickled ginger and scallions.

NUTRITION ESTIMATES (PER SERVING):
Calories: 510 | Protein: 28g | Carbs: 48g | Fat: 22g | Fiber: 1g

QUICK & EASY TIP: Use paper-thin beef cuts for ultra-fast cooking. Microwave rice saves even more time.

| 6. | **Tamagoyaki with Rice** |

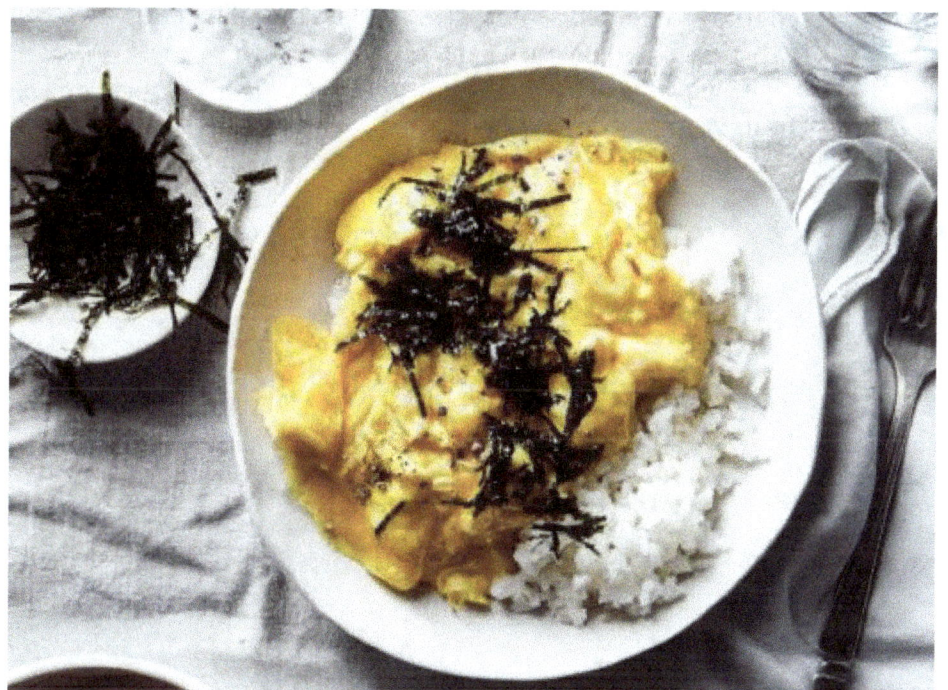

Prep Time: 3 minutes | Cook Time: 8 minutes | Makes: 2

Tamagoyaki, the sweet-savory rolled omelette, is a staple in Japanese bento and breakfast — but also makes a quick, protein-rich dinner when paired with rice. It's fluffy, delicate, and surprisingly satisfying.

INGREDIENTS:
- 4 large eggs
- 1 tbsp soy sauce
- 1 tsp sugar
- 1 tsp mirin
- 1 tsp oil
- 1 cup cooked Japanese rice
- Shredded nori or sesame seeds, for garnish

INSTRUCTIONS:
1. Beat eggs with soy sauce, sugar, and mirin.
2. Heat oil in a nonstick pan. Pour a thin layer of egg, roll it, then push to the side.
3. Repeat layering and rolling.
4. Slice the omelette and serve with rice. Garnish with nori or sesame seeds.

NUTRITION ESTIMATES (PER SERVING):
Calories: 410 | Protein: 20g | Carbs: 42g | Fat: 18g | Fiber: 1g

<u>*QUICK & EASY TIP:*</u> *A square tamagoyaki pan speeds up rolling, but a small round pan works fine too.*

7.	**Miso Glazed Cod**

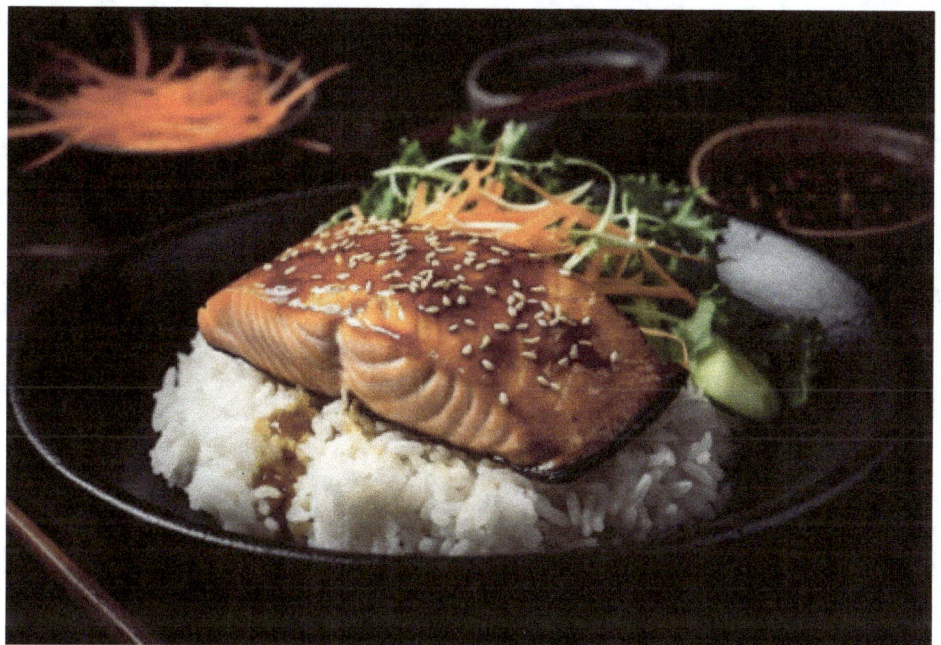

Prep Time: 4 minutes | Cook Time: 9 minutes | Makes: 2

This dish is inspired by Saikyo-yaki, a traditional Kyoto-style grilled fish marinated in sweet white miso. Its silky glaze and umami-rich flavor have made it a staple in upscale Japanese dining — but it's easy to replicate quickly at home using cod fillets.

INGREDIENTS:
- 2 cod fillets (approx. 120g each)
- 2 tbsp white miso paste
- 1 tbsp mirin
- 1 tsp soy sauce
- 1 tsp sugar
- 1 tsp oil
- Steamed rice, to serve

INSTRUCTIONS:
1. Mix miso, mirin, soy sauce, and sugar into a glaze.
2. Pat cod dry. Brush glaze onto each side.
3. Pan-fry fillets in oil over medium heat for 4–5 minutes per side until caramelized and cooked through.
4. Serve hot with rice.

NUTRITION ESTIMATES (PER SERVING):
Calories: 390 | Protein: 32g | Carbs: 10g | Fat: 24g | Fiber: 0g

QUICK & EASY TIP: *Use thin fillets for faster cooking. Preheat the pan to avoid sticking and save time.*

| 8. | Japanese Curry Udon |

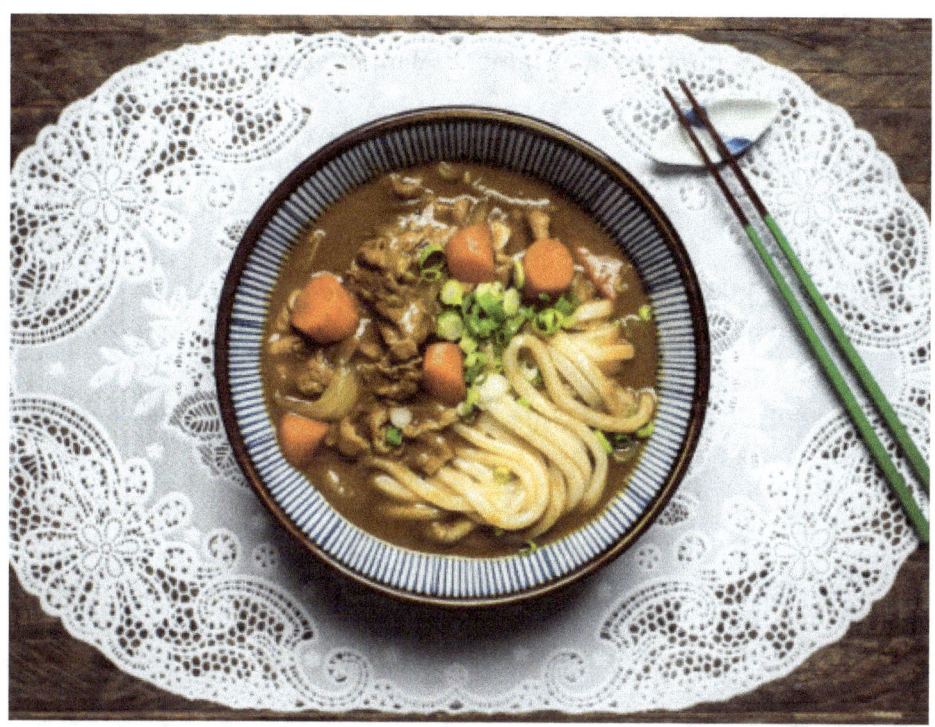

Prep Time: 5 minutes | Cook Time: 10 minutes | Makes: 2

Japanese Curry Udon is a soul-warming fusion of two beloved Japanese dishes: curry rice and udon noodle soup. Curry was introduced to Japan by the British in the late 1800s and was quickly adapted to local tastes, becoming a national favorite. Over time, it found its way into all kinds of comfort food—including this noodle version, which is especially popular in the colder months. Whether made from scratch or using instant curry roux, it's a fast, satisfying dish found in homes, cafeterias, and casual eateries across Japan.

INGREDIENTS:
- 1 pack frozen or fresh udon noodles
- ½ onion, thinly sliced
- ½ carrot, julienned
- 100g thin-sliced beef or tofu
- 1 Japanese curry cube (store-bought)
- 1 cup water
- 1 tsp oil
- Chopped green onions, to garnish

INSTRUCTIONS:
1. Sauté onion and carrot in oil for 2–3 minutes. Add beef or tofu.
2. Add water and curry cube. Simmer until dissolved (3–4 minutes).
3. Add udon noodles and simmer 2–3 minutes until heated through.
4. Garnish and serve.

NUTRITION ESTIMATES (PER SERVING):
Calories: 470 | Protein: 19g | Carbs: 54g | Fat: 20g | Fiber: 3g

<u>*QUICK & EASY TIP:*</u> *Use frozen pre-cooked udon and instant curry blocks to cut down prep to near zero.*

MEDITERRANEAN DINNERS

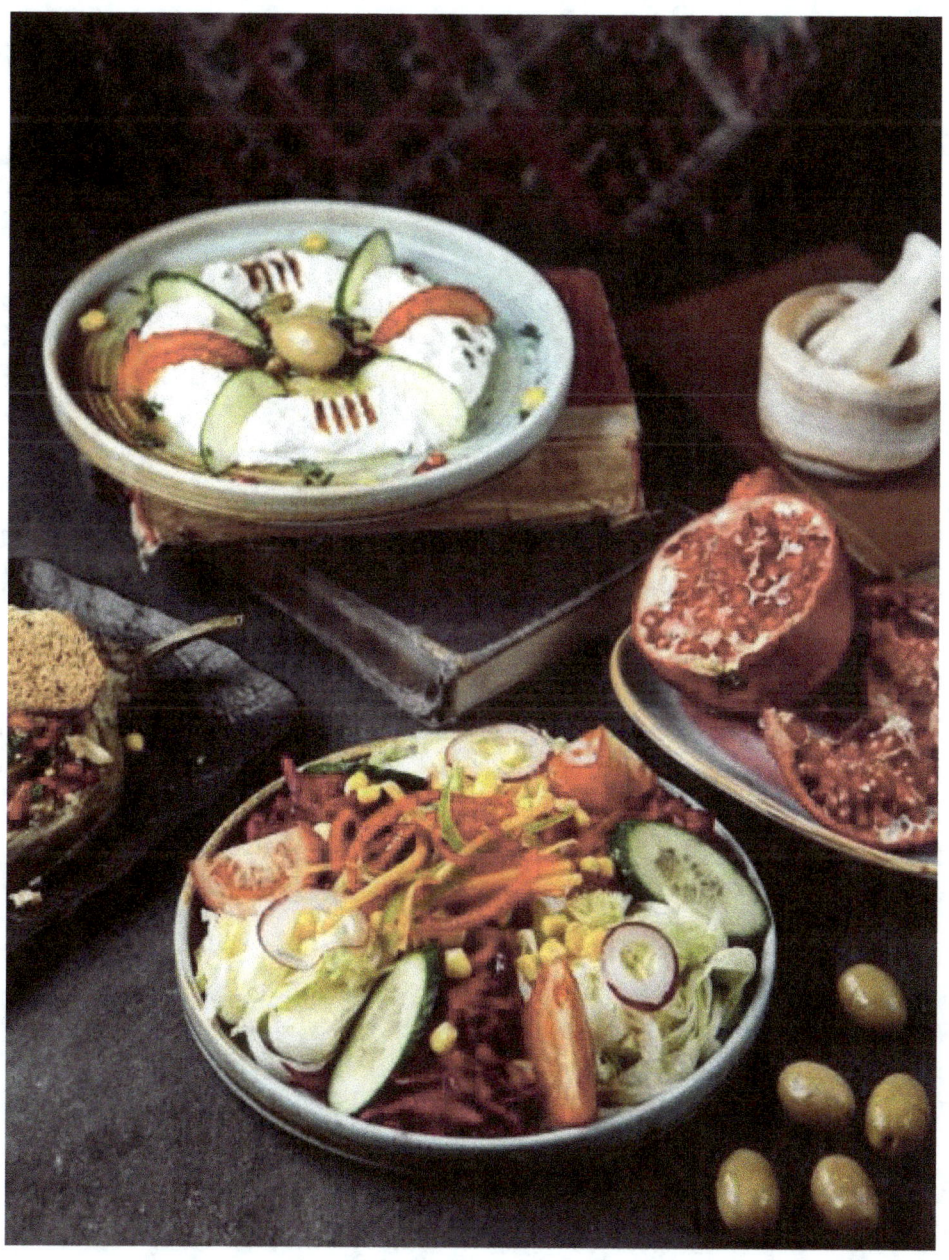

| 9. | **Pasta with Spinach and Walnut Pesto** |

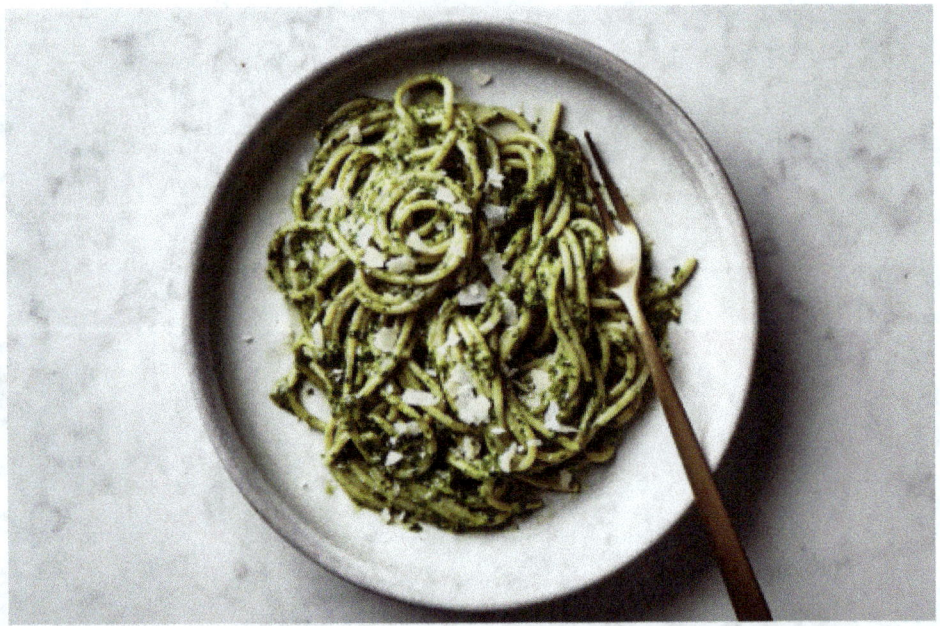

Prep Time: 10 min | Cook Time: 15 min | Makes: 4 servings

Pesto has long roots in Mediterranean cuisine, particularly from Italy's Ligurian coast. This vibrant, dairy-free version swaps basil for spinach and cheese for nutritional yeast, creating a nutritious and satisfying dish. It's a flavorful, plant-based dinner that comes together quickly and easily for busy weeknights.

INGREDIENTS:
- 8 oz gluten-free pasta
- 2 cups fresh spinach
- ½ cup walnuts
- ¼ cup olive oil
- 2 cloves garlic
- ¼ cup nutritional yeast
- Juice of 1 lemon
- Salt and pepper to taste

INSTRUCTIONS:
1. Cook pasta according to package instructions. Drain and set aside.
2. In a food processor, blend spinach, walnuts, garlic, and nutritional yeast until finely chopped.

3. With processor running, drizzle in olive oil until a smooth pesto forms. Add lemon juice and pulse to combine.
4. Season with salt and pepper.
5. Toss pesto with cooked pasta until well coated.
6. Serve warm.

NUTRITION ESTIMATES (PER SERVING):
Calories: 320 | Protein: 8g | Carbs: 40g | Fat: 15g | Fiber: 4g

QUICK & EASY TIP: *Use pre-washed spinach and pre-chopped walnuts to save time. The pesto can be made in advance and stored for up to 3 days.*

| 10. | Herb Shrimp Pasta |

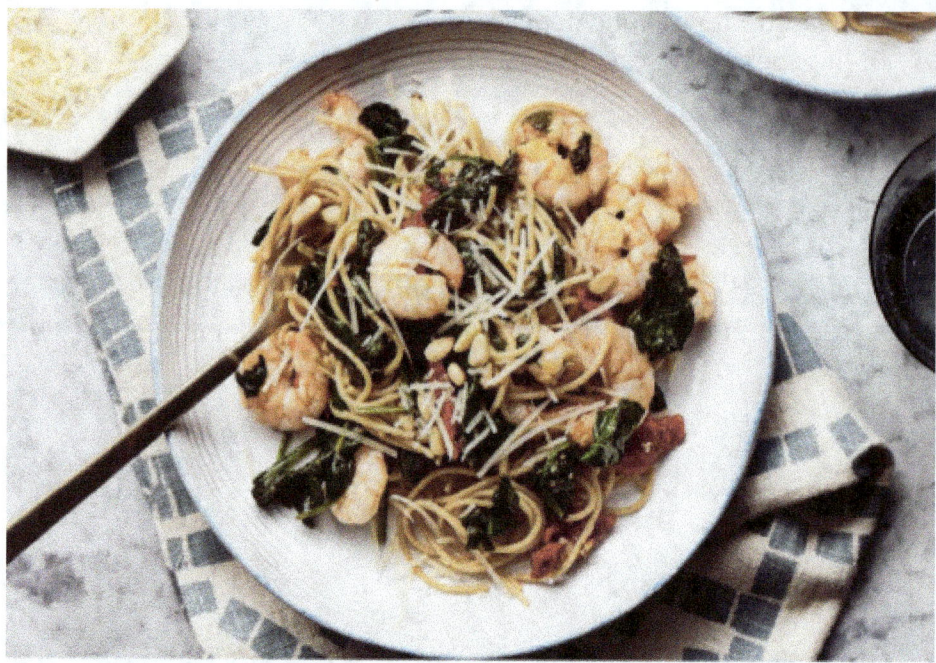

Prep Time: 10 min | Cook Time: 15 min | Makes: 4 servings

Mediterranean cuisine often celebrates simplicity with bold flavors, and this herb shrimp pasta is a perfect example. The combination of dried herbs and fresh lemon captures the coastal essence of southern Europe, where seafood and fresh herbs reign supreme. It's fast, flavorful, and satisfying.

INGREDIENTS:
- 8 oz (225 g) pasta (such as penne or spaghetti)
- 1 tablespoon olive oil
- 1 pound (450 g) large shrimp, peeled and deveined
- 3 cloves garlic, minced
- 1 teaspoon dried basil
- 1 teaspoon dried oregano
- ½ teaspoon dried thyme
- ¼ teaspoon red pepper flakes (optional, for a touch of heat)
- Salt and pepper to taste
- ¼ cup fresh parsley, chopped
- ¼ cup fresh basil, chopped
- Juice of 1 lemon
- 2 tablespoons grated Parmesan cheese (optional)

INSTRUCTIONS:
1. Cook pasta according to package instructions. Drain and set aside.
2. Heat olive oil in a large skillet over medium heat.
3. Add shrimp and cook 2–3 minutes per side until pink and opaque.
4. Add garlic, dried herbs, and red pepper flakes. Cook 1–2 minutes until fragrant.
5. Season with salt and pepper.
6. Add pasta to the skillet and toss to combine.
7. Remove from heat. Stir in parsley, basil, and lemon juice.
8. Serve warm with Parmesan if desired.

NUTRITION ESTIMATES (PER SERVING):
Calories: 350 | Protein: 20g | Carbs: 40g | Fat: 12g | Fiber: 3g

QUICK & EASY TIP: Use frozen, pre-peeled shrimp and pre-chopped herbs for quicker prep.

11. Pesto Zucchini Noodles with Grilled Chicken

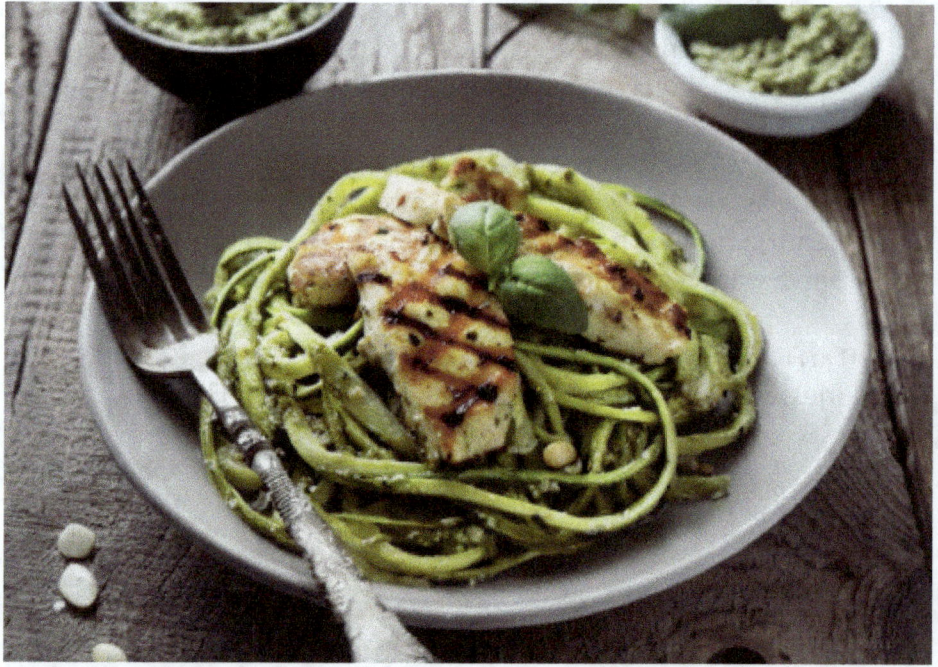

Prep Time: 15 min | Cook Time: 15 min | Makes: 4 servings

This light yet flavorful dish draws from Italian traditions with a healthy twist. Replacing traditional pasta with zucchini noodles makes it perfect for low-carb or gluten-free diners, while still delivering the beloved flavor of classic pesto and grilled chicken.

INGREDIENTS:
- 4 medium zucchinis, spiralized into noodles
- 2 tbsp olive oil
- 2 grilled chicken breasts, sliced
- ¼ cup store-bought pesto
- ¼ cup pine nuts, toasted (optional)
- Salt and pepper to taste

INSTRUCTIONS:
1. Heat olive oil in a skillet over medium heat.
2. Sauté zucchini noodles for 3–4 minutes until just tender.
3. Toss with pesto and season with salt and pepper.
4. Plate zucchini noodles. Top with sliced grilled chicken.
5. Sprinkle with pine nuts if using.
6. Serve immediately.

NUTRITION ESTIMATES (PER SERVING):
Calories: 320 | Protein: 30g | Carbs: 18g | Fat: 18g | Fiber: 3g

<u>QUICK & EASY TIP</u>: Use pre-cooked grilled chicken and store-bought spiralized zucchini for maximum speed.

> **12.**   **Chicken Souvlaki with Tzatziki**

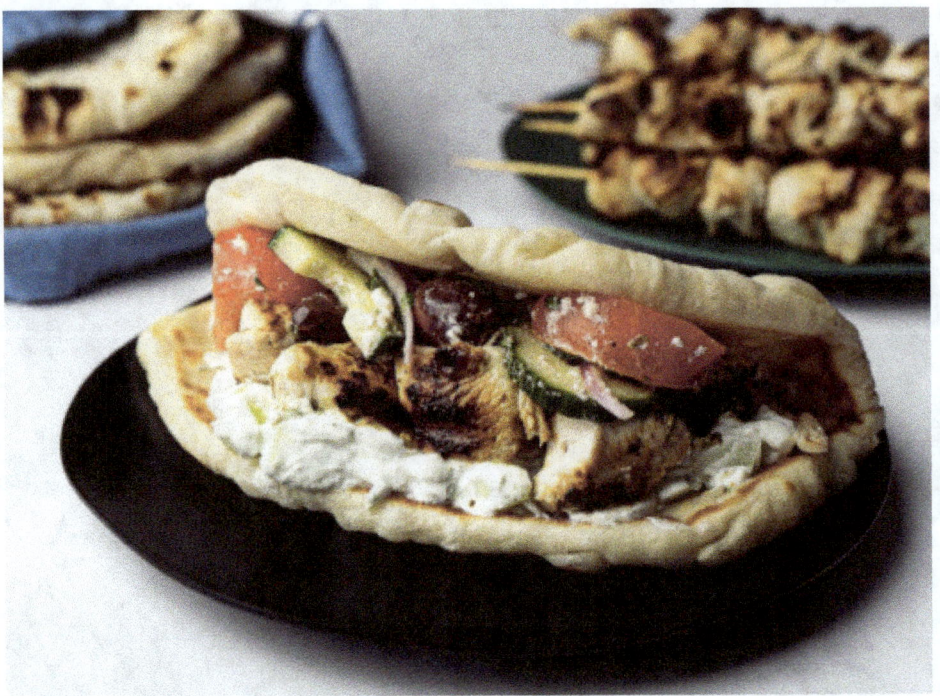

Prep Time: 5 minutes | Cook Time: 9 minutes | Makes: 2

Souvlaki dates back to ancient Greece, where skewered meats were cooked over open flames as early as the 5th century BCE. Today, it remains one of Greece's most iconic street foods — quick, flavorful, and widely enjoyed. This version skips the skewers and grill for a speedy stovetop sear, while still capturing the essence of the dish. Paired with cool, creamy tzatziki — a yogurt and cucumber sauce with roots in Ottoman and Balkan cuisine — this meal brings the warmth of the Mediterranean to your table in minutes.

INGREDIENTS:
- 200g boneless chicken breast or thigh, cut into chunks
- 1 tbsp olive oil
- 1 tsp dried oregano
- ½ tsp garlic powder
- Salt and pepper, to taste
- ½ cup Greek yogurt
- ¼ cucumber, grated
- 1 clove garlic, minced
- 1 tsp lemon juice

INSTRUCTIONS:
1. Mix chicken with olive oil, oregano, garlic powder, salt, and pepper.
2. Sear in a pan for 7–9 minutes until cooked through.
3. Combine yogurt, cucumber, garlic, and lemon juice to make tzatziki.
4. Serve chicken with tzatziki on the side, with pita or salad if desired.

NUTRITION ESTIMATES (PER SERVING):
Calories: 410 | Protein: 36g | Carbs: 6g | Fat: 26g | Fiber: 1g

QUICK & EASY TIP: Use pre-cut chicken and grate the cucumber while the chicken cooks to save time.

| 13. | **Tuna and White Bean Salad** |

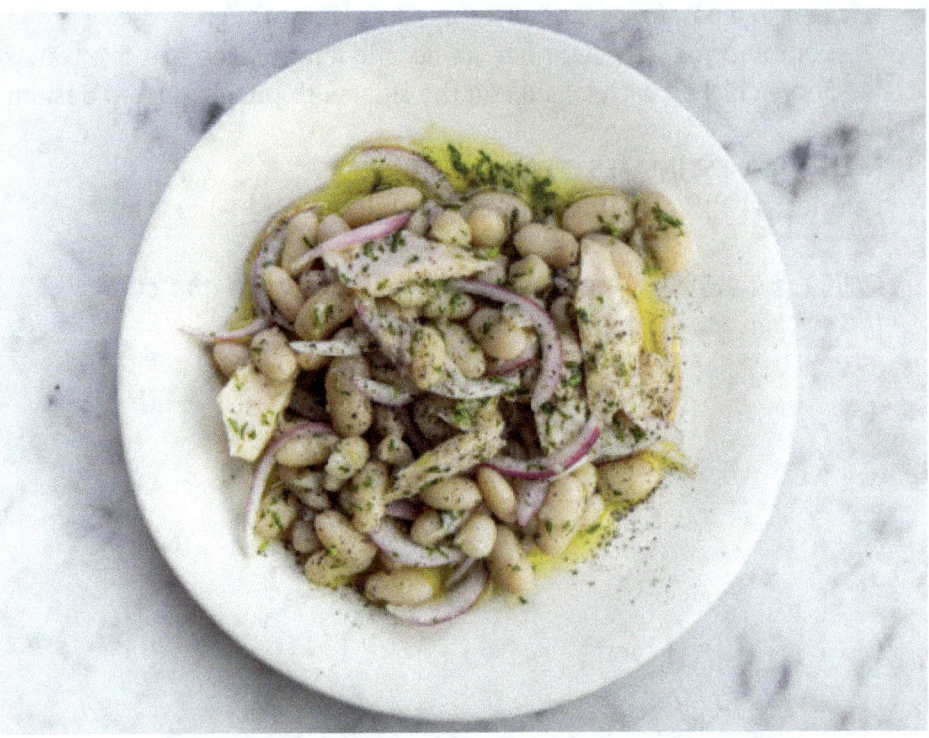

Prep Time: 7 minutes | Cook Time: None | Makes: 2

Sailors along the Mediterranean coast, especially in Italy and Spain, traditionally relied on preserved tuna and beans for quick, protein-rich meals at sea. This classic combination is still a pantry staple across Southern Europe, offering a refreshing, no-cook dinner that's perfect for warm-weather evenings or busy weeknights.

INGREDIENTS:
- 1 can (150g) tuna in olive oil, drained
- 1 cup canned white beans (cannellini), rinsed
- 1 small red onion, thinly sliced
- 1 cup cherry tomatoes, halved
- 2 tbsp chopped parsley
- 2 tbsp olive oil
- 1 tbsp lemon juice
- Salt and pepper, to taste

INSTRUCTIONS:
1. Combine tuna, beans, onion, tomatoes, and parsley in a bowl.

2. Drizzle with olive oil and lemon juice. Season with salt and pepper.
3. Toss gently and serve chilled or at room temperature.

NUTRITION ESTIMATES (PER SERVING):
Calories: 430 | Protein: 29g | Carbs: 22g | Fat: 26g | Fiber: 6g

QUICK & EASY TIP: Use canned ingredients and pre-chopped herbs for ultimate speed — no cooking required.

14. Grilled Eggplant and Halloumi Stacks

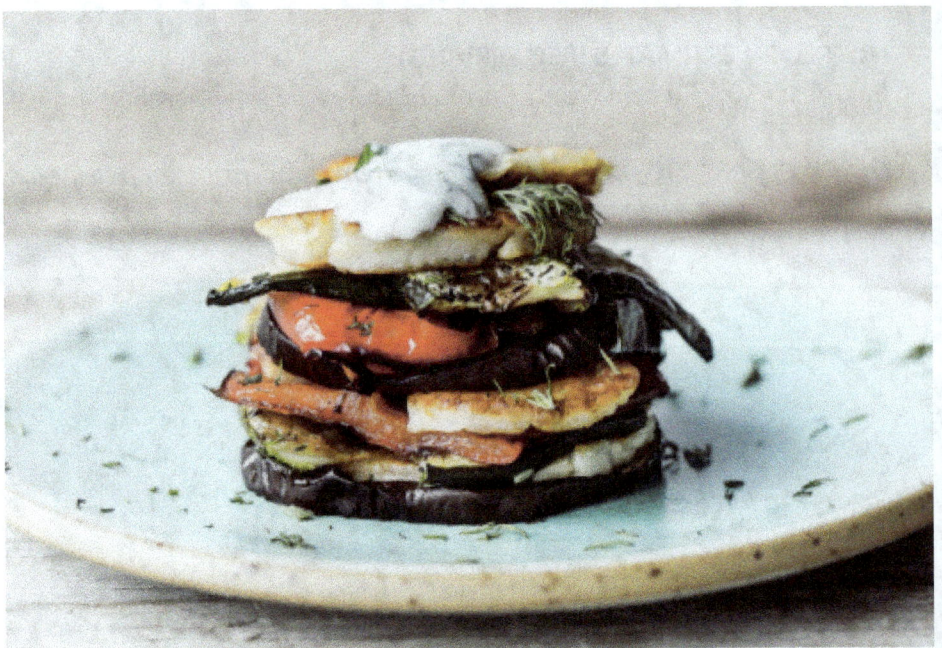

Prep Time: 5 minutes | Cook Time: 8 minutes | Makes: 2

Eggplant, or aubergine, has been cherished across the Middle East and Mediterranean for centuries—once even believed to have mystical properties in ancient Arabic medicine. Halloumi, a brined cheese from Cyprus, dates back to the Byzantine era and was traditionally stored in mint to keep it fresh. Together, these ingredients form a timeless vegetarian dish that's as flavorful as it is quick.

INGREDIENTS:
- 1 small eggplant, sliced into rounds
- 150g halloumi cheese, sliced
- 1 medium tomato, sliced
- 1 tbsp olive oil
- ½ tsp dried thyme or za'atar
- Fresh mint or basil, for garnish

INSTRUCTIONS:

1. Slice the eggplant into ½-inch rounds and lightly pat them dry with a paper towel to reduce moisture. Brush both sides with olive oil and sprinkle with dried thyme or za'atar for added flavor.

2. Heat a grill pan or nonstick skillet over medium-high heat. Add the eggplant slices in a single layer and grill for 3–4 minutes per side until golden brown and tender. Remove and set aside.
3. In the same pan, grill the halloumi slices for about 2–3 minutes per side until they're golden and lightly crisp on the outside. Avoid overcrowding the pan to get an even sear.
4. To assemble the stacks, layer one slice of eggplant, one tomato slice, and one slice of halloumi. Repeat for 2–3 layers per stack, depending on thickness and portion size.
5. Garnish the stacks with fresh mint or basil leaves. Serve warm as a light dinner or appetizer, with a drizzle of olive oil or a side of yogurt dip if desired.

NUTRITION ESTIMATES (PER SERVING):
Calories: 450 | Protein: 20g | Carbs: 12g | Fat: 36g | Fiber: 5g

QUICK & EASY TIP: *Use a grill pan to cook everything at once. No peeling or salting eggplant needed.*

15. Garlic Shrimp with Lemon Couscous

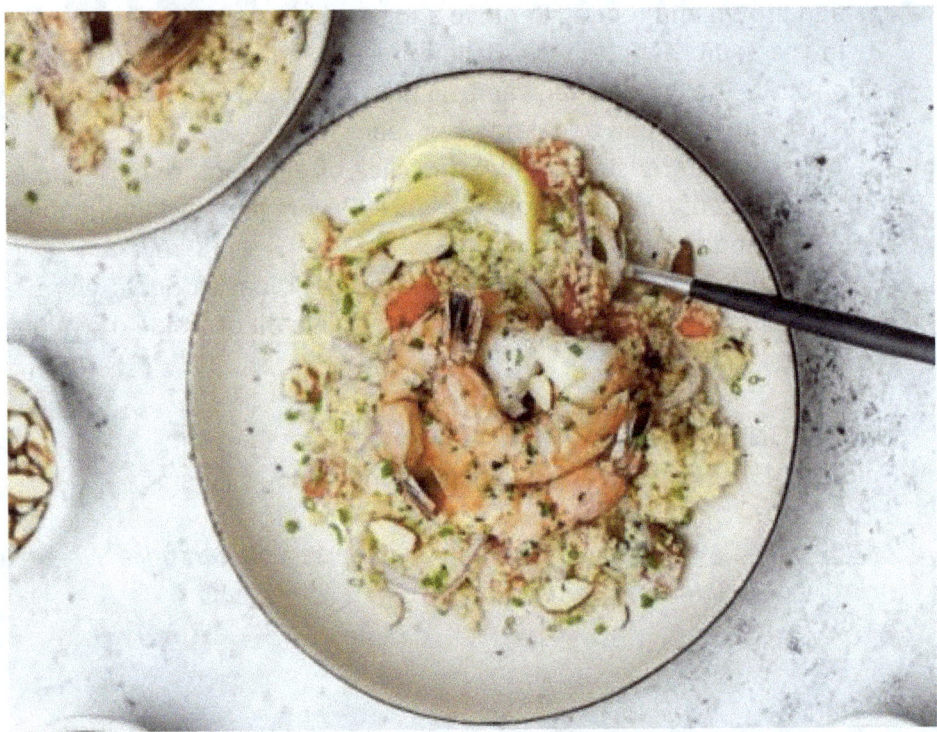

Prep Time: 5 minutes | Cook Time: 10 minutes | Makes: 2

Inspired by the sun-soaked coasts of Spain and Morocco, this dish combines bold Iberian flavors with a North African staple. Shrimp sautéed in garlic and paprika reflects classic Spanish tapas, while fluffy couscous—a dish dating back to Berber tribes over a thousand years ago—offers a quick, satisfying base. The lemony twist ties both worlds together in a zesty, modern way.

INGREDIENTS:
- 200g shrimp, peeled and deveined
- 1 tbsp olive oil
- 2 cloves garlic, minced
- ½ tsp smoked paprika
- 1 cup instant couscous
- ¾ cup hot vegetable broth or water
- 1 tbsp lemon juice
- Fresh parsley, chopped

INSTRUCTIONS:

1. In a bowl, combine couscous with hot broth. Cover and let sit 5 minutes. Fluff with a fork.
2. Meanwhile, sauté garlic in olive oil. Add shrimp and paprika.
3. Cook for 4–5 minutes until pink.
4. Stir lemon juice into couscous.
5. Serve shrimp over couscous and sprinkle with parsley.

NUTRITION ESTIMATES (PER SERVING):
Calories: 470 | Protein: 30g | Carbs: 38g | Fat: 22g | Fiber: 2g

QUICK & EASY TIP: Use frozen pre-peeled shrimp and instant couscous to cut active cooking time in half.

16. Lemon Pasta with Spinach and Feta

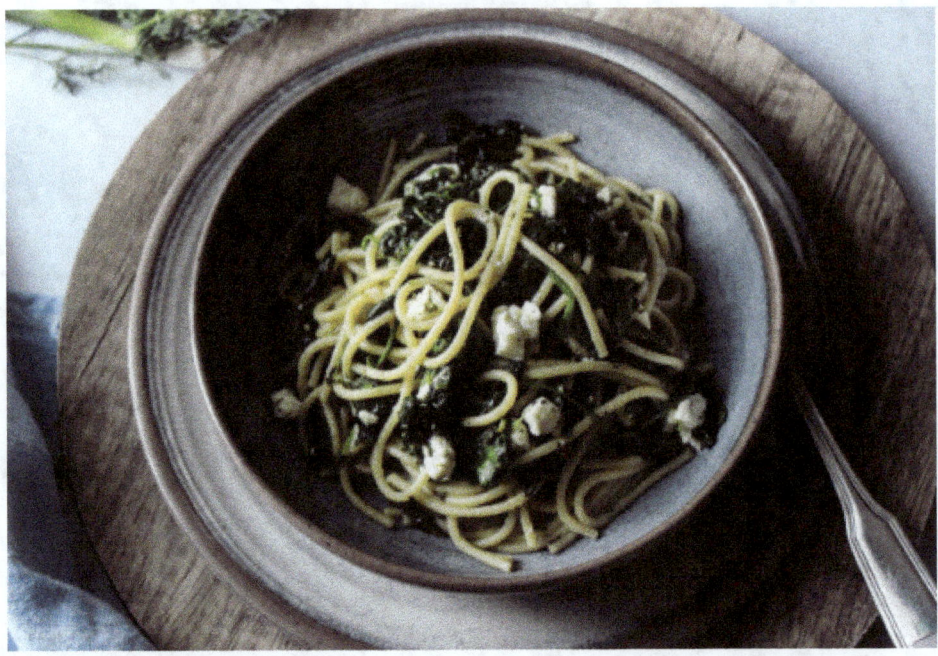

Prep Time: 4 minutes | Cook Time: 10 minutes | Makes: 2

Mediterranean cuisine has long prized the harmony of simple, seasonal ingredients. In Greece, feta cheese has been produced for over 6,000 years and remains a national treasure, while lemon and olive oil are central to both Greek and Italian culinary traditions. This dish draws from that legacy—combining vibrant lemon, briny feta, and silky pasta into a meal that captures the essence of sun-drenched coastal cooking. It's fast, fresh, and deeply rooted in centuries of flavor tradition.

INGREDIENTS:
- 150g spaghetti or angel hair pasta
- 2 tbsp olive oil
- 2 cloves garlic, thinly sliced
- 2 cups baby spinach
- ½ lemon, juiced
- ½ cup crumbled feta cheese
- Salt and black pepper, to taste

INSTRUCTIONS:

1. Bring a pot of salted water to a boil and cook pasta until al dente, about 6–8 minutes for spaghetti or 3–4 minutes for angel hair. Drain and reserve ¼ cup of pasta water.
2. While pasta cooks, heat olive oil in a large skillet over medium heat. Add sliced garlic and sauté for 30–60 seconds until fragrant but not browned.
3. Add baby spinach to the skillet and stir for 1–2 minutes until just wilted.
4. Add the cooked pasta to the skillet along with lemon juice and reserved pasta water. Toss well to coat.
5. Stir in crumbled feta, season with salt and black pepper, and toss until cheese is just starting to melt and everything is well combined.
6. Serve immediately, garnished with extra feta or lemon zest if desired.

NUTRITION ESTIMATES (PER SERVING):
Calories: 480 | Protein: 16g | Carbs: 52g | Fat: 24g | Fiber: 4g

QUICK & EASY TIP: *Use angel hair pasta for faster boiling. Pre-washed spinach saves prep time.*

17. Chickpea and Olive Skillet with Harissa

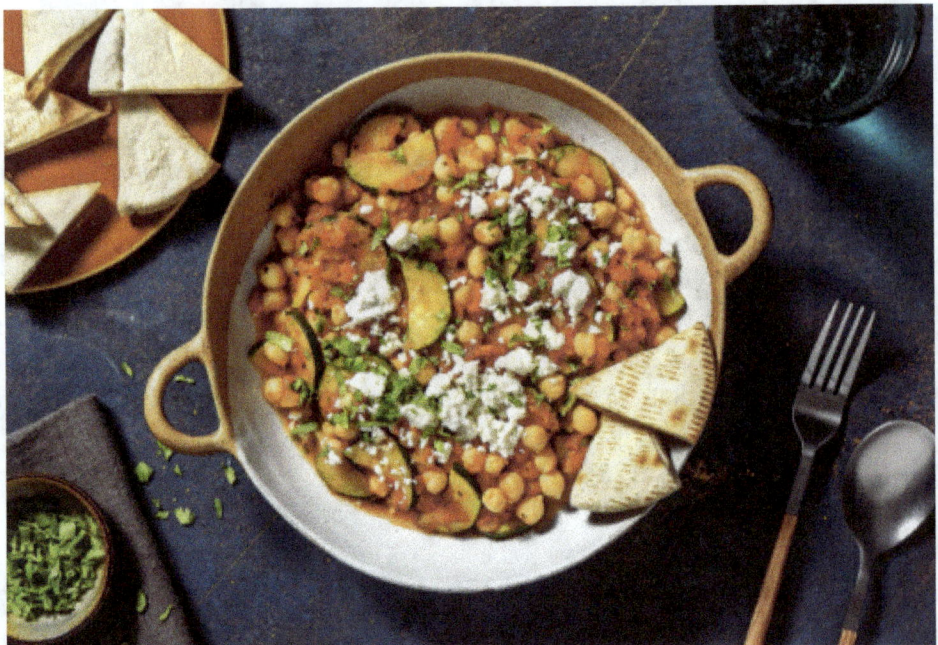

Prep Time: 5 minutes | Cook Time: 8 minutes | Makes: 2

Chickpeas, also known as garbanzo beans, have been a staple across North Africa and the Middle East for thousands of years. Combined with olives—another ancient Mediterranean ingredient—and the fiery North African chili paste harissa, this dish captures the essence of Maghrebi home cooking. It's fast, filling, and delivers bold flavor in every bite—no meat required.

INGREDIENTS:
- 1 can chickpeas (drained and rinsed)
- ¼ cup pitted green or black olives
- 1 small red onion, sliced
- ½ cup crushed tomatoes
- 1 tbsp harissa paste
- 1 tbsp olive oil
- Salt and lemon juice, to taste
- 2 tbsp crumbled feta cheese
- Fresh cilantro or parsley, to garnish
- Flatbread crisps, for serving

INSTRUCTIONS:

1. Sauté onion in olive oil for 2 minutes. Add chickpeas, olives, and harissa.
2. Stir in crushed tomatoes and simmer for 5–6 minutes until thickened.
3. Season with salt and a splash of lemon juice. Top with feta and garnish with herbs.
4. Serve warm with flatbread crisps.

NUTRITION ESTIMATES (PER SERVING):
Calories: 420 | Protein: 14g | Carbs: 36g | Fat: 24g | Fiber: 9g

<u>QUICK & EASY TIP:</u> Use canned chickpeas and jarred harissa to minimize prep. Serve with bread or couscous if desired.

18. Herb-Crusrted Lamb Chops

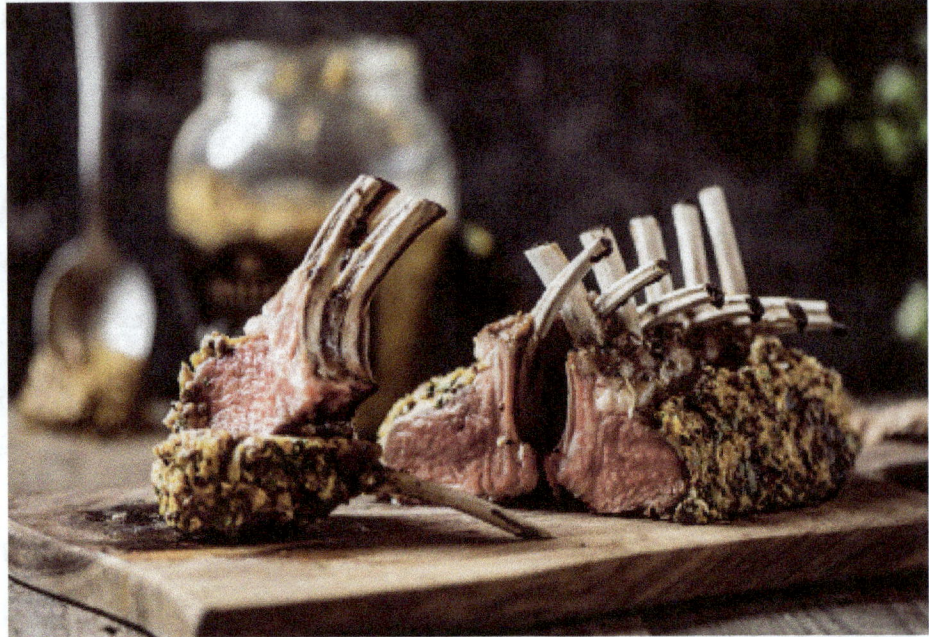

Prep Time: 10 min | Cook Time: 15 min | Makes: 2

Lamb has been a prized meat in Mediterranean cuisine for millennia, dating back to ancient Greece and Rome, where it was often reserved for festive occasions and religious feasts. In regions like Provence and coastal Greece, it's traditionally prepared with local herbs—such as rosemary and thyme—grown in abundance. This herb-crusted version blends those regional influences into a dish that's quick enough for a weeknight meal, yet rich in flavor and heritage.

INGREDIENTS:
- 4 lamb chops
- 2 tbsp olive oil
- 1 tbsp fresh rosemary, chopped
- 1 tbsp fresh thyme, chopped
- 2 cloves garlic, minced
- ½ tsp salt
- ¼ tsp black pepper

INSTRUCTIONS:
1. Preheat oven to 375°F (190°C).
2. Mix olive oil, rosemary, thyme, garlic, salt, and pepper in a bowl.
3. Rub the herb mixture onto both sides of the lamb chops.

4. Heat a skillet over medium-high heat and sear the lamb chops for 2–3 minutes per side until browned.
5. Transfer the skillet to the oven and bake for 8–10 minutes, or until desired doneness.

NUTRITION ESTIMATES (PER SERVING):
Calories: 400 | Protein: 40g | Carbs: 1g | Fat: 28g | Fiber: 0g

QUICK & EASY TIP: *For quicker prep, use pre-chopped herbs or a ready-made herb blend. Pair with roasted vegetables or couscous for a full meal.*

AMERICAN DINNERS

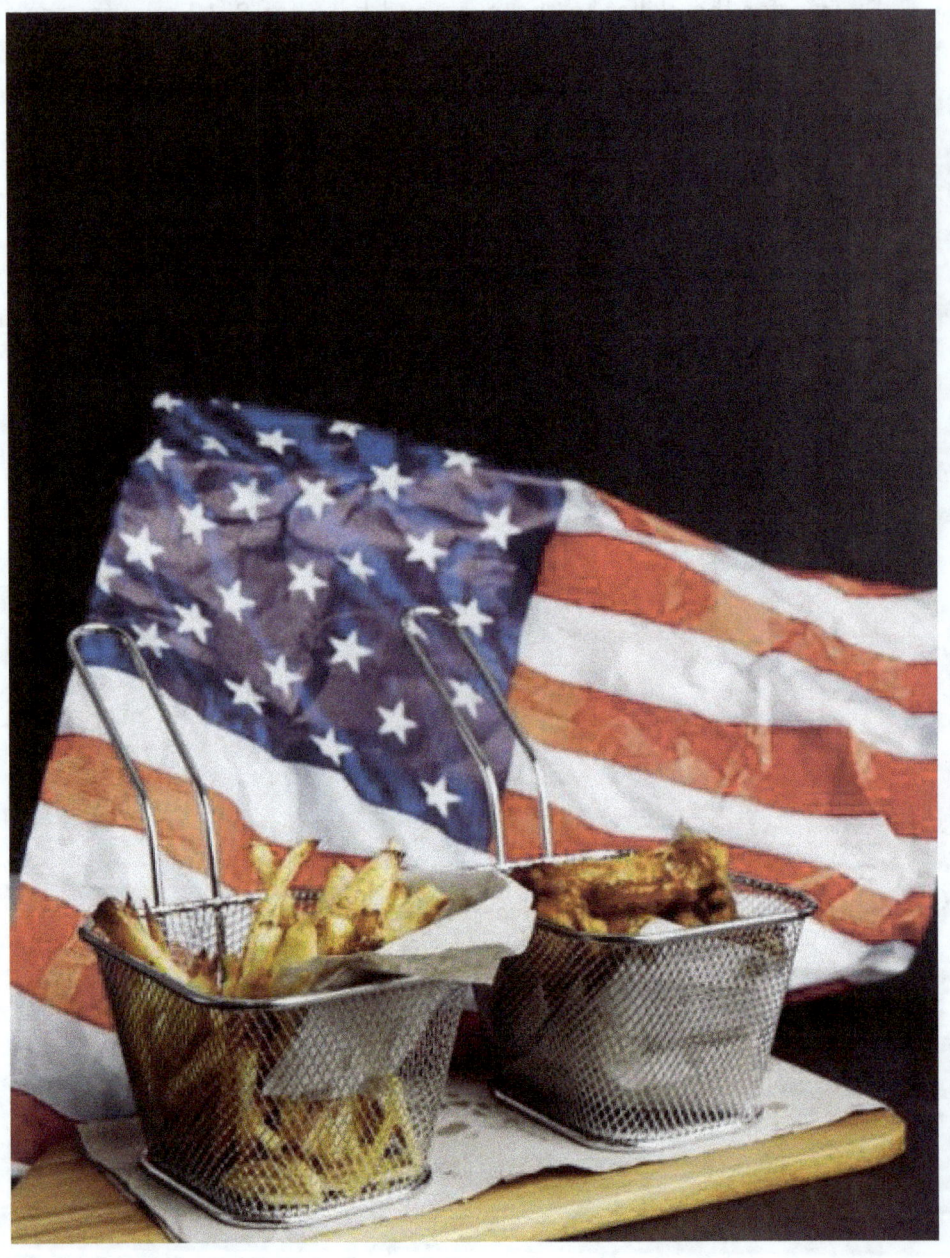

19. Almond-Crusted Salmon with Salad

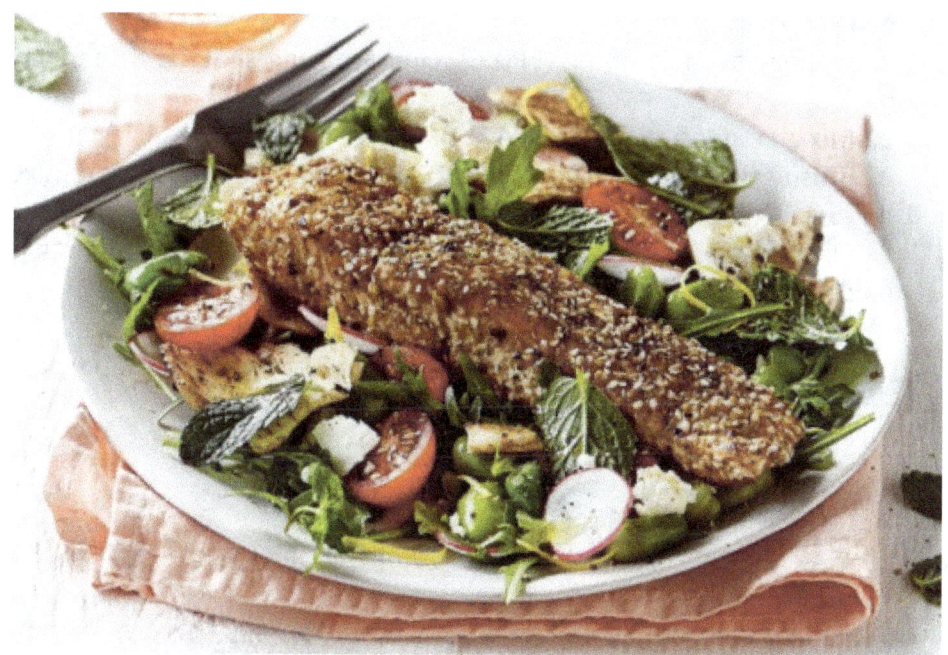

Prep Time: 10 min | Cook Time: 15 min | Makes: 4 servings

Almond-crusted salmon is a modern take on classic American baked fish, inspired by health-conscious trends from California cuisine. The use of nuts in place of breadcrumbs reflects a shift toward whole foods and gluten-free alternatives—without sacrificing texture or flavor.

INGREDIENTS:
FOR THE ALMOND-CRUSTED SALMON:
- 4 salmon fillets (about 6 oz each)
- ½ cup almonds, finely chopped
- 2 tablespoons almond flour or whole wheat flour
- 1 tablespoon olive oil
- 1 tablespoon Dijon mustard
- Salt and pepper to taste

FOR THE SALAD:
- 4 cups mixed greens (such as spinach, arugula, or lettuce)
- 1 cup cherry tomatoes, halved
- ½ cucumber, sliced
- ¼ cup red onion, thinly sliced
- 1 avocado, sliced
- 2 tablespoons olive oil
- 1 tablespoon lemon juice

- Salt and pepper to taste

INSTRUCTIONS:
1. Preheat oven to 400°F (200°C). Line a baking sheet with parchment paper.
2. Mix almonds and almond flour in a bowl.
3. Brush salmon with olive oil and Dijon mustard. Press almond mixture on top.
4. Place salmon on the baking sheet and bake for 12–15 minutes until golden and cooked through.
5. Toss greens, tomatoes, cucumber, onion, and avocado in a bowl.
6. Drizzle with olive oil and lemon juice, season with salt and pepper, and toss to combine.
7. Serve salmon alongside the salad.

NUTRITION ESTIMATES (PER SERVING):
Calories: 400 | Protein: 30g | Carbs: 12g | Fat: 28g | Fiber: 5g

<u>QUICK & EASY TIP:</u> Use pre-chopped almonds and store-bought salad mix to cut prep time in half.

| 20. | Lemon Herb Grilled Chicken |

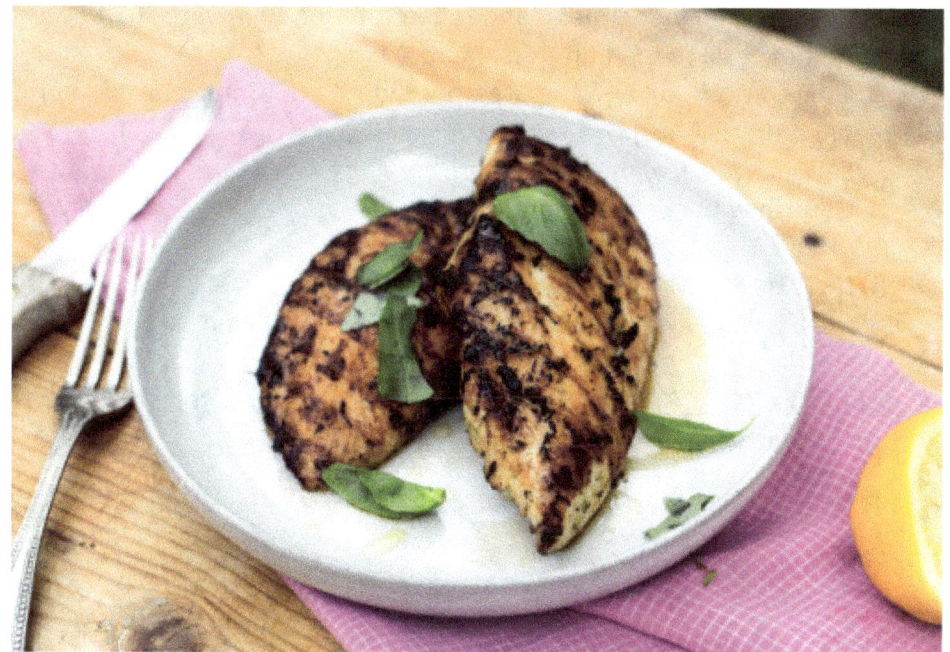

Prep Time: 10 minutes | Cook Time: 15 minutes | Makes: 4 servings

Grilled chicken with lemon and herbs has roots in American backyard barbecues, but its flavor profile draws heavily from Mediterranean traditions. It became a popular low-fat protein choice during the fitness boom of the 1980s and remains a staple in health-forward American kitchens.

INGREDIENTS:
- 4 boneless, skinless chicken breasts
- 2 tbsp olive oil
- Juice of 1 lemon
- Zest of 1 lemon
- 2 garlic cloves, minced
- 1 tsp dried oregano
- 1 tsp dried thyme
- ½ tsp ground black pepper
- ½ tsp salt
- Fresh parsley, chopped, for garnish

INSTRUCTIONS:

1. Whisk olive oil, lemon juice, zest, garlic, oregano, thyme, salt, and pepper in a bowl.
2. Coat chicken in marinade and refrigerate for 30 minutes to 4 hours.
3. Preheat grill to medium-high heat.
4. Grill chicken for 6–7 minutes per side or until internal temperature reaches 165°F (74°C).
5. Let rest for a few minutes before serving.
6. Garnish with chopped parsley.

NUTRITION ESTIMATES (PER SERVING):
Calories: 280 | Protein: 32g | Carbs: 2g | Fat: 16g | Fiber: 0.5g

QUICK & EASY TIP: *Marinate earlier in the day for a faster dinner rush. Also works well cold in salads or wraps.*

21. Seared Scallops with Spinach

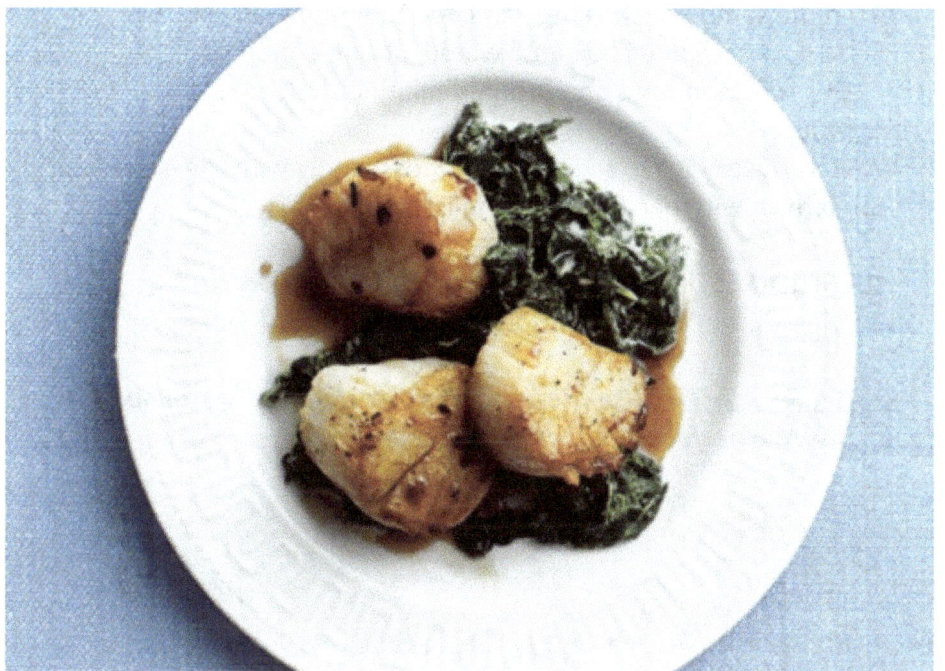

Prep Time: 10 min | Cook Time: 10 min | Makes: 2 servings

Seared scallops are a classic American coastal delicacy, especially prominent in New England cuisine. Their quick cooking time and elegant presentation have made them a favorite for fine dining and weeknight meals alike. Paired with garlicky spinach, this dish balances indulgence with simplicity.

INGREDIENTS:
- 8 large sea scallops (about 1 pound or 450 g)
- 1 tablespoon olive oil
- Salt and pepper to taste
- 2 cups fresh spinach leaves
- 2 cloves garlic, minced
- 1 tablespoon lemon juice
- ¼ cup chicken broth or water
- 1 tablespoon chopped fresh parsley (for garnish)

INSTRUCTIONS:
1. Pat scallops dry with paper towels and season with salt and pepper.
2. Heat olive oil in a skillet over medium-high heat.

3. Add scallops without crowding. Sear 2–3 minutes per side until golden and opaque. Remove and set aside.
4. In the same skillet, sauté garlic for 1 minute until fragrant.
5. Add spinach and cook until wilted, about 2 minutes.
6. Stir in lemon juice and broth, deglazing the pan. Simmer 1–2 minutes to reduce.
7. Return scallops to the skillet and toss gently with the spinach mixture.
8. Garnish with parsley and serve immediately.

NUTRITION ESTIMATES (PER SERVING):
Calories: 250 | Protein: 25g | Carbs: 5g | Fat: 15g | Fiber: 2g

<u>*QUICK & EASY TIP:*</u> *Use pre-washed spinach and dry scallops thoroughly to ensure a perfect sear in under 10 minutes.*

22. Cod with Sautéed Spinach

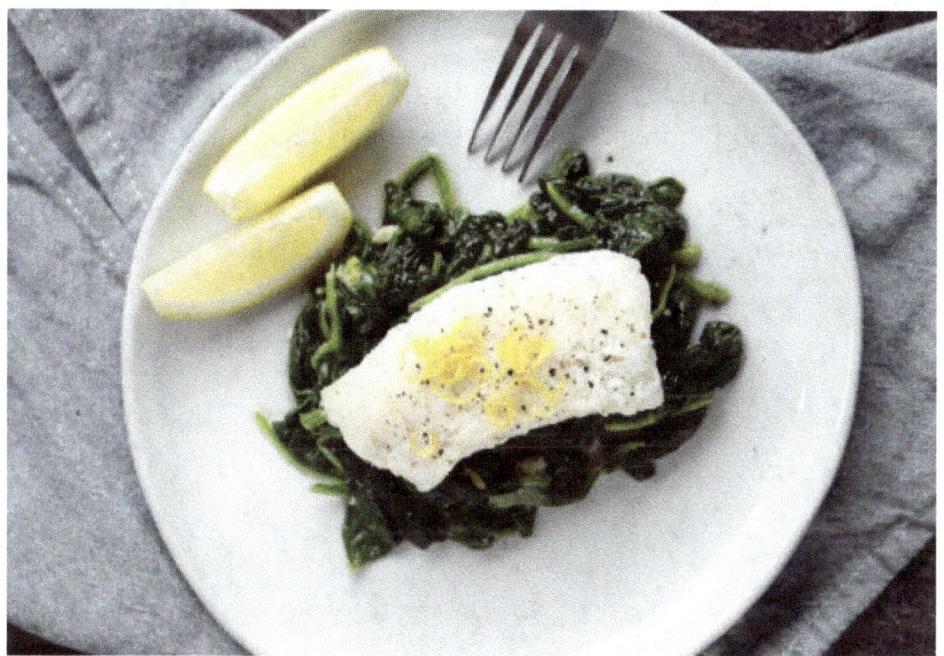

Prep Time: 10 min | Cook Time: 15 min | Makes: 4 servings

A staple of classic American home cooking, cod is a mild, flaky white fish that's both versatile and nutritious. This dish pairs it with garlicky sautéed spinach for a light, wholesome meal inspired by coastal New England, where seafood has long played a starring role in regional cuisine.

INGREDIENTS:
- 4 cod fillets (about 6 oz each)
- 2 tablespoons olive oil, divided
- 2 garlic cloves, minced
- 1 lemon, sliced
- 6 cups fresh spinach, washed and dried
- Salt and pepper to taste

INSTRUCTIONS:
1. Season cod fillets with salt and pepper. Heat 1 tbsp olive oil in a large skillet over medium heat.
2. Add cod and cook for 3–4 minutes per side, until opaque and flaky. Remove from skillet and keep warm.
3. In the same skillet, heat remaining 1 tbsp olive oil. Sauté garlic for 1 minute until fragrant.

4. Add spinach and cook, stirring, for 3–4 minutes until wilted. Season with salt and pepper.
5. Serve spinach alongside cod fillets and garnish with lemon slices.

NUTRITION ESTIMATES (PER SERVING):
Calories: 250 | Protein: 32g | Carbs: 4g | Fat: 12g | Fiber: 2g

<u>*QUICK & EASY TIP:*</u> *Use pre-washed spinach and frozen cod fillets (thawed) to reduce prep time.*

23. Sweet Potato Noodles with Spinach

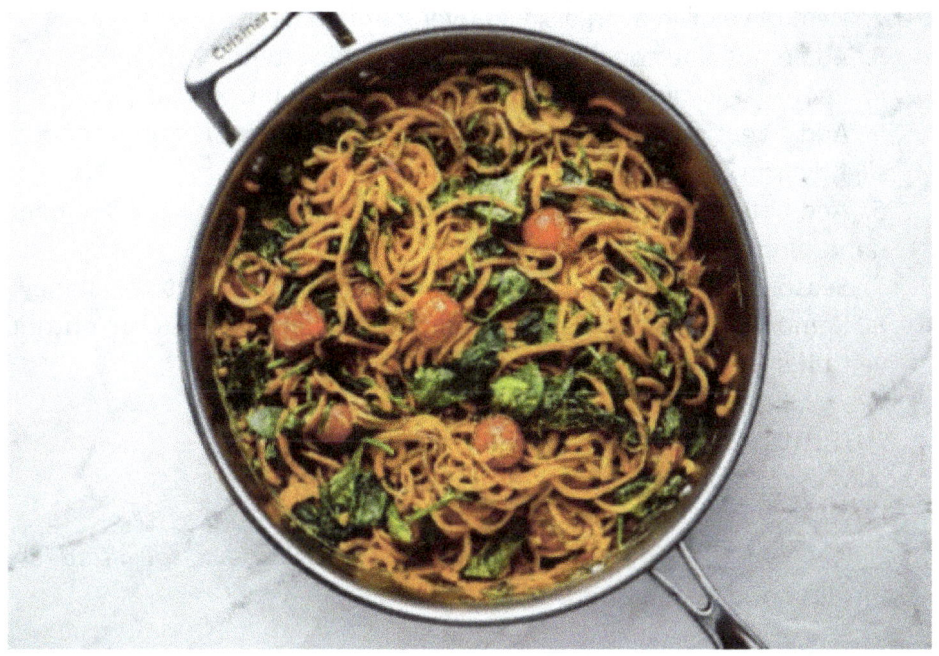

Prep Time: 10 min | Cook Time: 15 min | Makes: 4 servings

This vibrant, veggie-packed dish is a modern take on classic comfort food, blending wholesome ingredients with Mediterranean-style flavors. Spiralized sweet potatoes provide a gluten-free noodle alternative, while spinach and herbs boost the nutritional punch. It's a perfect plant-based meal that's as colorful as it is nourishing.

INGREDIENTS:
- 2 medium sweet potatoes, spiralized into noodles
- 1 tablespoon olive oil
- 1 small onion, diced
- 2 cloves garlic, minced
- 1 red bell pepper, sliced
- 1 cup baby spinach
- ½ cup cherry tomatoes, halved
- 1 teaspoon dried oregano
- ½ teaspoon dried basil
- Salt and pepper to taste
- 2 tablespoons chopped fresh parsley (for garnish)
- Optional: ¼ cup crumbled feta cheese or nutritional yeast (for a dairy-free option)

INSTRUCTIONS:
1. Spiralize the sweet potatoes using a spiralizer or julienne peeler.
2. Heat olive oil in a large skillet over medium heat.
3. Add onion and cook for 3–4 minutes until softened.
4. Stir in garlic and cook for 1 minute until fragrant.
5. Add sweet potato noodles and cook for 5–7 minutes until tender but slightly firm.
6. Add bell pepper, spinach, and cherry tomatoes. Cook for 3–4 minutes until spinach wilts.
7. Season with oregano, basil, salt, and pepper. Stir well to combine.
8. Remove from heat, garnish with parsley, and add feta or nutritional yeast if desired.

NUTRITION ESTIMATES (PER SERVING):
Calories: 180 | Protein: 5g | Carbs: 30g | Fat: 6g | Fiber: 5g

<u>*QUICK & EASY TIP:*</u> *Save time by purchasing pre-spiralized sweet potatoes and bagged baby spinach.*

| 24. | Steak Bites with Garlic Butter |

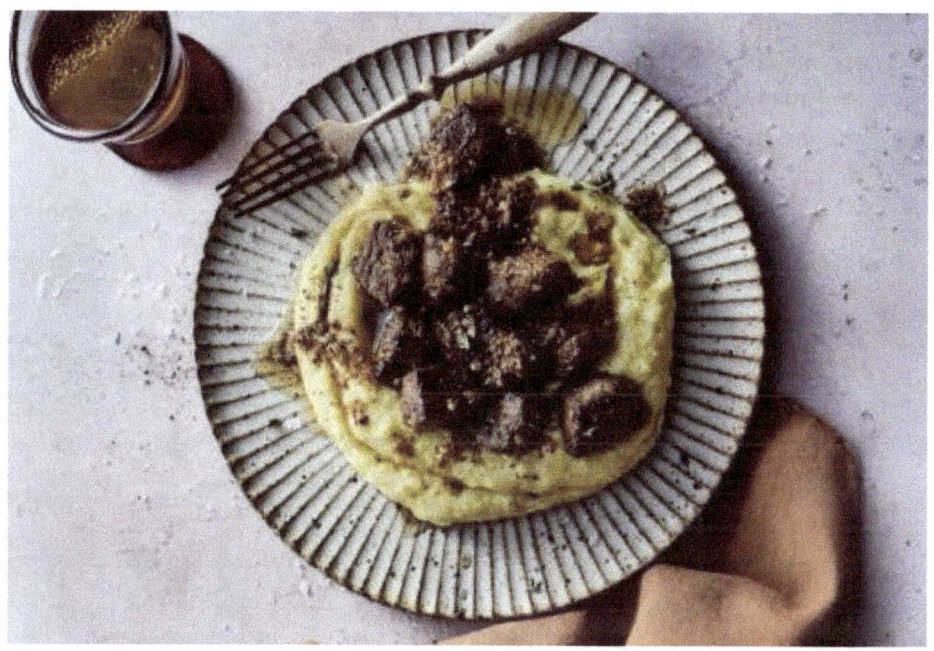

Prep Time: 4 minutes | Cook Time: 10 minutes | Makes: 2

Garlic butter steak bites are a modern take on American steakhouse fare—hearty, fast, and full of bold flavor. This stovetop version captures all the richness of a grilled steak in bite-sized pieces, ideal for busy nights. Fun fact: The sizzling steak bite trend actually gained popularity through viral online videos showcasing the irresistible combo of browned beef and melted garlic butter—now a staple in home kitchens across the U.S.

INGREDIENTS:
- 250g sirloin or ribeye steak, cut into 1-inch cubes
- 1 tbsp olive oil
- 1 tbsp butter
- 2 cloves garlic, minced
- Salt and black pepper, to taste
- 1 tbsp chopped fresh parsley

INSTRUCTIONS:
1. Pat steak cubes dry with a paper towel to ensure better browning.
2. Season generously with salt and black pepper.
3. Heat olive oil in a large skillet over high heat until just smoking.
4. Add steak cubes in a single layer without crowding the pan. Let sear undisturbed for 2–3 minutes to develop a golden-brown crust.

5. Flip steak bites and cook for another 2 minutes to sear the other sides.
6. Reduce heat to medium-low. Add butter and minced garlic. Stir continuously for 1–2 minutes to coat the steak and prevent the garlic from burning.
7. Once the garlic is fragrant and the steak is cooked to your liking, remove from heat.
8. Sprinkle with fresh parsley and serve immediately with rice, mashed potatoes, or a side salad.

NUTRITION ESTIMATES (PER SERVING):
Calories: 410 | Protein: 35g | Carbs: 1g | Fat: 30g | Fiber: 0g

QUICK & EASY TIP: *Cut steak ahead of time and use a hot skillet to reduce cook time.*

25. BBQ Chicken Wraps

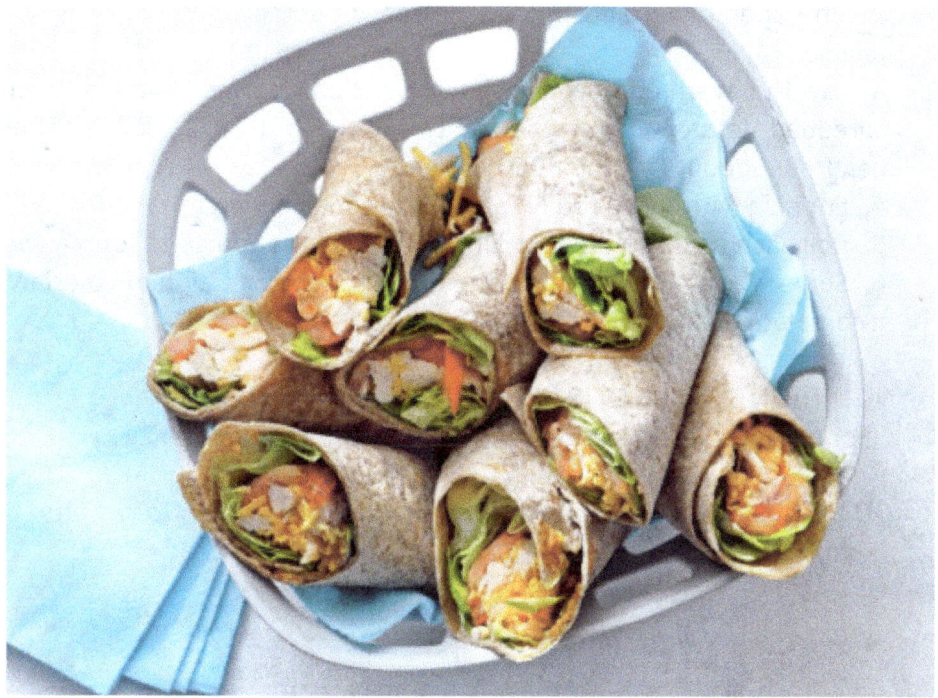

Prep Time: 5 minutes | Cook Time: 8 minutes | Makes: 2

Barbecue has deep roots in American culinary tradition, tracing back to Southern pitmasters and backyard cookouts. While traditional BBQ is slow-smoked and time-intensive, this wrap captures the bold, smoky-sweet essence in minutes. With tender shredded chicken, tangy sauce, crunchy slaw, and melty cheese all wrapped in a soft tortilla, it's your favorite cookout—no grill required.

INGREDIENTS:
- 1 cooked chicken breast, shredded (or 200g rotisserie chicken)
- ¼ cup BBQ sauce
- 2 large flour tortillas
- ½ cup shredded lettuce or slaw mix
- ¼ red onion, thinly sliced
- ½ cup shredded cheddar cheese

INSTRUCTIONS:
1. In a medium skillet over medium heat, add the cooked chicken and pour in the BBQ sauce. Stir well to coat all the pieces evenly. Cook for 2–3 minutes, stirring occasionally, until the chicken is heated through and the sauce is bubbling.

2. While the chicken warms, heat the tortillas in a dry skillet over medium heat for about 15–20 seconds on each side, or wrap them in a damp paper towel and microwave for 20–30 seconds until warm and pliable.
3. Lay the warmed tortillas flat on a clean surface. Add a layer of shredded lettuce down the center of each tortilla, followed by a generous spoonful of the BBQ chicken.
4. Sprinkle with sliced red onion and shredded cheese.
5. Roll each tortilla tightly, tucking in the sides as you go to form a wrap.
6. Serve warm with your favorite dipping sauce or a side of coleslaw for a complete meal.

NUTRITION ESTIMATES (PER SERVING):
Calories: 470 | Protein: 32g | Carbs: 34g | Fat: 24g | Fiber: 2g

QUICK & EASY TIP: *Use pre-cooked or rotisserie chicken to cut prep time in half.*

26. Classic Patty Melt

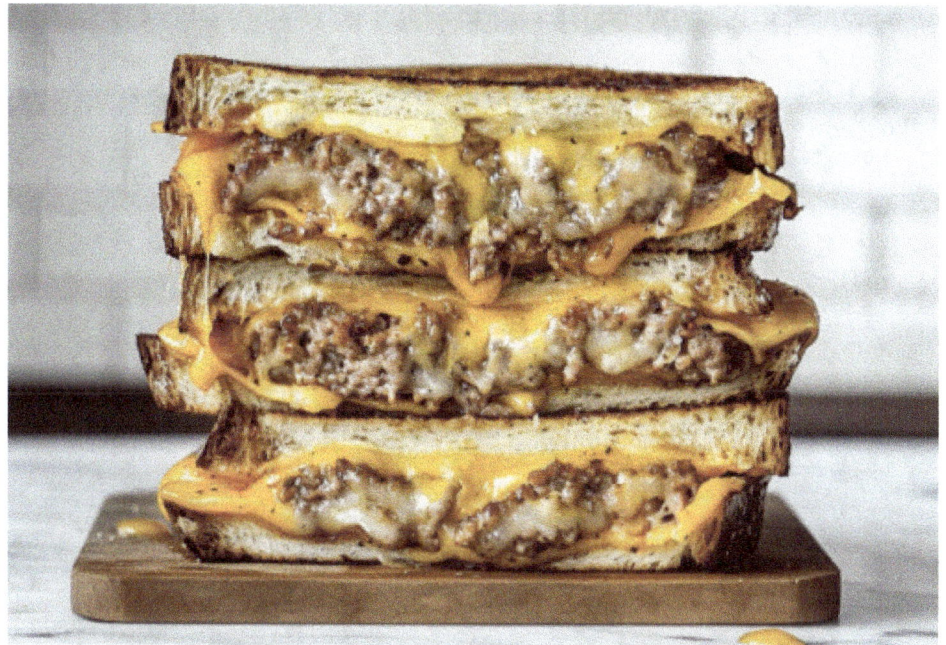

Prep Time: 4 minutes | Cook Time: 10 minutes | Makes: 2

A staple of American diners since the 1940s, the patty melt is a cross between a grilled cheese and a burger. It features a seasoned beef patty, caramelized onions, and melted cheese sandwiched between slices of toasted rye or sourdough.

INGREDIENTS:
- 250g ground beef
- ½ small onion, thinly sliced
- 4 slices rye or sourdough bread
- 2 slices Swiss or cheddar cheese
- 1 tbsp butter
- Salt and pepper, to taste

INSTRUCTIONS:
1. Shape ground beef into 2 thin patties. Season with salt and pepper.
2. In a skillet, cook onions in butter for 3–4 minutes until soft. Remove.
3. Cook patties for 3–4 minutes per side until browned and cooked through.
4. Assemble each sandwich: bread, cheese, patty, onions, more cheese, bread.
5. Toast in the skillet 1–2 minutes per side until golden and melted.

NUTRITION ESTIMATES (PER SERVING):
Calories: 610 | Protein: 32g | Carbs: 28g | Fat: 42g | Fiber: 2g

QUICK & EASY TIP: *Use pre-sliced cheese and pre-sliced bread for faster assembly. Onions can be pre-cooked and stored for the week.*

| 27. | Cheesy Chicken Quesadillas |

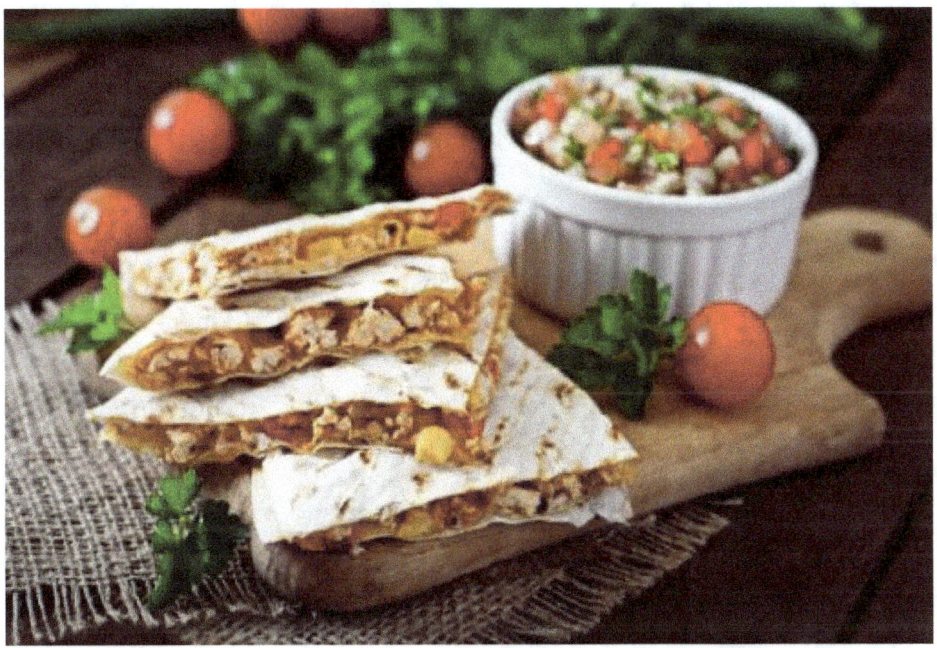

Prep Time: 5 minutes | Cook Time: 8 minutes | Makes: 2

Quesadillas are a beloved cross-cultural dish in the U.S., especially in the Southwest, where Tex-Mex influence is strong. This cheesy chicken version is pan-fried to crisp perfection, stuffed with flavorful filling, and endlessly customizable.

INGREDIENTS:
- 2 large flour tortillas
- 1 cup shredded cooked chicken
- ½ cup shredded cheddar or Monterey Jack cheese
- 2 tbsp salsa or taco sauce
- 1 tbsp olive oil
- Optional: sour cream or guacamole, to serve

INSTRUCTIONS:
1. In a medium mixing bowl, combine the shredded cooked chicken, grated cheese, and salsa. Stir until all the ingredients are evenly mixed.
2. Lay out the tortillas on a clean surface. Spoon the chicken mixture onto one half of each tortilla, spreading it evenly but leaving a small border around the edge to prevent overflow. Fold the other half of the tortilla over the filling to form a half-moon shape.

3. Heat a skillet over medium heat and add a small amount of oil. Once hot, place the folded quesadillas in the skillet (working in batches if needed). Cook for 3–4 minutes per side, pressing gently with a spatula, until both sides are golden brown and crispy, and the cheese has melted.
4. Transfer the quesadillas to a cutting board and let them rest for a minute before slicing into wedges.
5. Serve warm with your favorite dips such as sour cream, guacamole, or extra salsa.

NUTRITION ESTIMATES (PER SERVING):
Calories: 480 | Protein: 30g | Carbs: 28g | Fat: 28g | Fiber: 2g

<u>QUICK & EASY TIP:</u> Use leftover chicken or rotisserie meat. Grate cheese ahead and store for quick use.

| 28. | **Chili Cheese Dogs** |

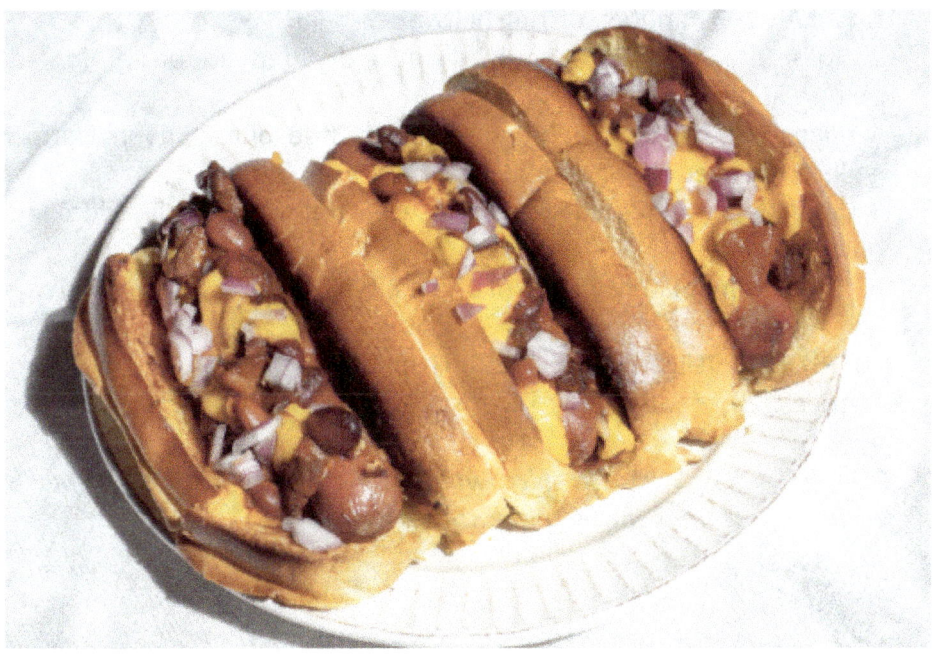

Prep Time: 5 minutes | Cook Time: 10 minutes | Makes: 2

Chili cheese dogs are an iconic symbol of American casual dining, with roots tracing back to the early 20th century when hot dog stands began topping franks with hearty chili to attract hungry workers. Popularized by ballparks, diners, and drive-ins across the U.S., this indulgent combination of savory hot dog, meaty chili, and melty cheese delivers pure comfort in every bite. Quick, filling, and endlessly customizable, it's a nostalgic favorite that's always a crowd-pleaser.

INGREDIENTS:
- 2 beef or chicken hot dogs
- 2 hot dog buns
- ½ cup canned or leftover chili
- ¼ cup shredded cheddar cheese
- 1 tbsp chopped onion (optional)

INSTRUCTIONS:
1. Heat a skillet over medium heat. Add the hot dogs and cook for 3–4 minutes, turning occasionally, until warmed through and slightly browned. Alternatively, microwave them for 1 minute.

2. In a small saucepan, warm the chili over low heat for 3–4 minutes, stirring occasionally. You can also microwave it in a microwave-safe bowl for about 1–2 minutes, stirring halfway through.
3. Toast the hot dog buns lightly in a dry pan or toaster for added texture, if desired.
4. Place the cooked hot dogs in the toasted buns. Spoon warm chili generously over each hot dog.
5. Sprinkle shredded cheddar cheese on top of the chili. Add chopped onion if using.
6. Serve immediately while hot and melty.

NUTRITION ESTIMATES (PER SERVING):
Calories: 520 | Protein: 24g | Carbs: 32g | Fat: 34g | Fiber: 2g

QUICK & EASY TIP: *Use microwave-safe steps to cut cook time even further. Toast buns for texture boost.*

MEXICAN DINNERS

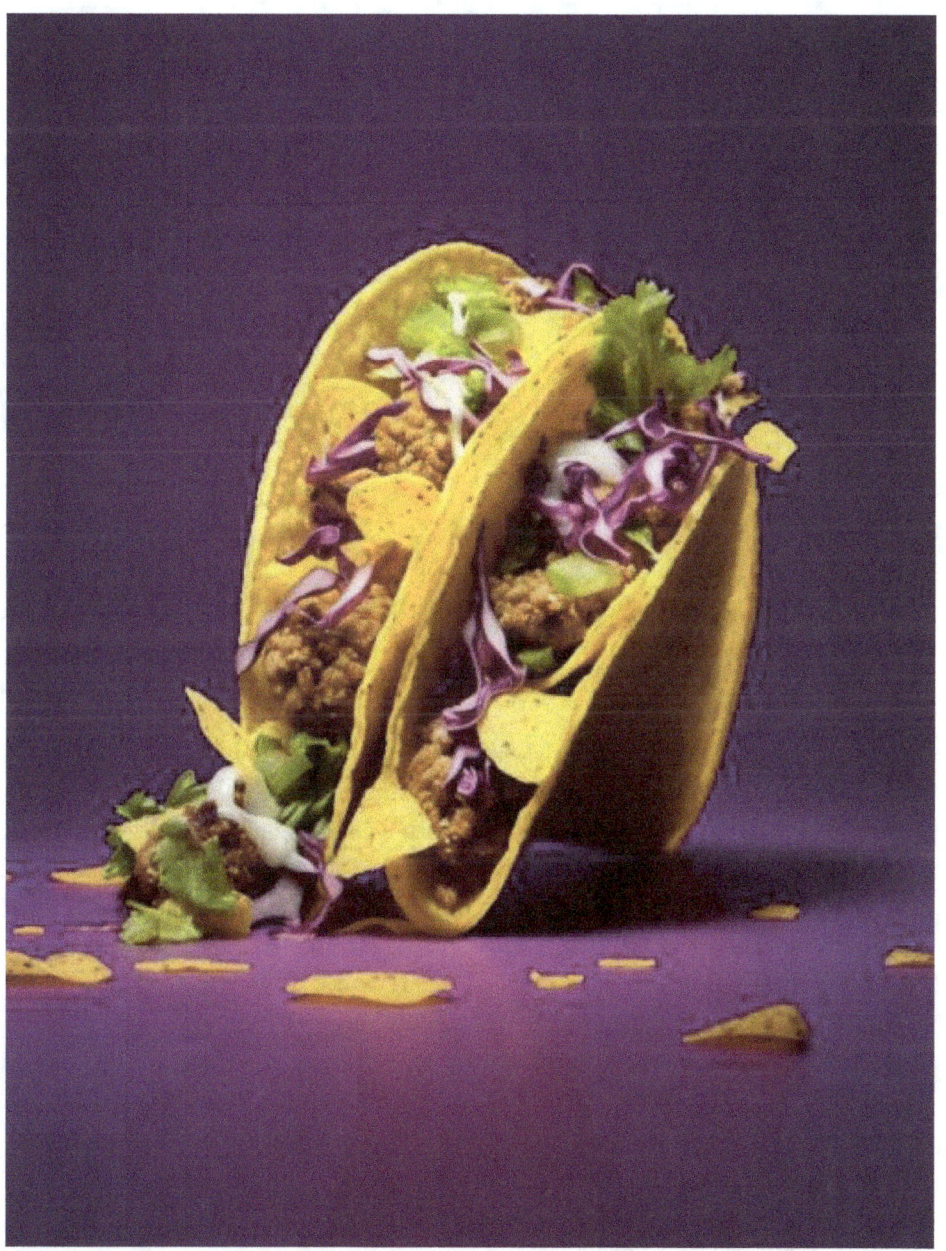

29. Fish Tacos with Pico de Gallo

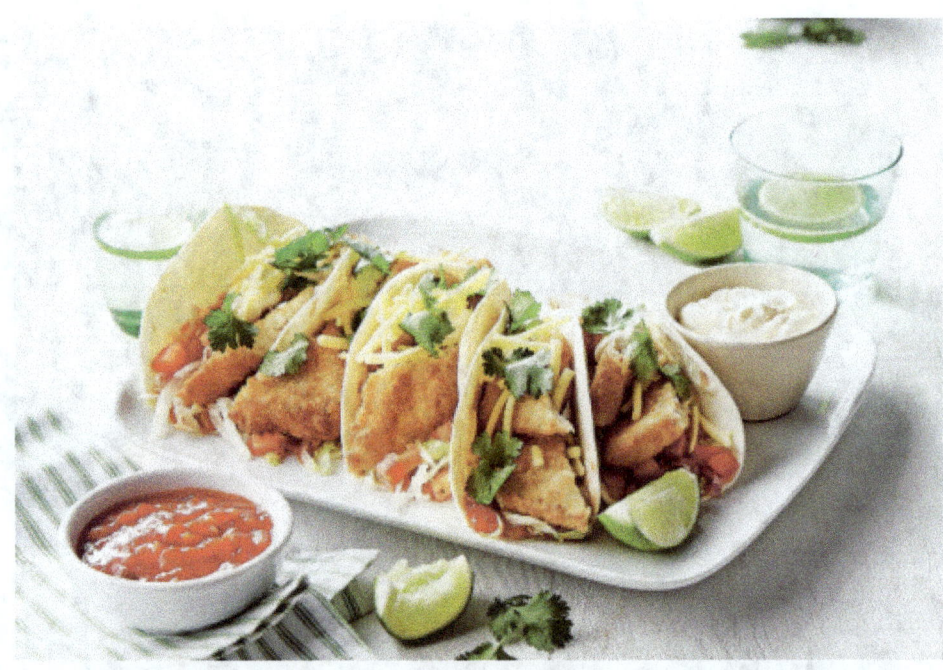

Prep Time: 5 min | Cook Time: 10 min | Makes: 4 servings

Fish tacos are a coastal Mexican staple, particularly popular in Baja California. Originally made with battered and fried fish, this lighter version uses pan-seared white fish and fresh pico de gallo, a salsa of chopped tomatoes, cilantro, and lime. It's a delicious balance of spice, crunch, and citrus, all wrapped in warm corn tortillas — a true reflection of Mexico's vibrant street food culture.

INGREDIENTS:
FOR THE FISH:
- 1 lb (450 g) firm white fish (like cod or tilapia), cut into bite-sized pieces
- 2 tbsp olive oil
- 1 tsp ground cumin
- ½ tsp smoked paprika
- ½ tsp chili powder
- ½ tsp dried oregano
- ¼ tsp salt
- ¼ tsp black pepper
- Juice of 1 lime

FOR SERVING:
- 1 cup store-bought pico de gallo

- 8 small corn tortillas
- 1 cup pre-shredded lettuce or cabbage
- Lime wedges (for garnish)
- Fresh cilantro (optional, for garnish)

INSTRUCTIONS:
1. Mix olive oil, cumin, paprika, chili powder, oregano, salt, pepper, and lime juice in a bowl. Add fish and toss to coat.
2. Heat a non-stick skillet over medium heat. Cook fish for 2–3 minutes per side, until golden and flaky.
3. Warm tortillas in a dry skillet or microwave.
4. Layer lettuce or cabbage on each tortilla. Top with cooked fish and spoonfuls of store-bought pico de gallo.
5. Garnish with lime wedges and cilantro if desired. Serve immediately.

NUTRITION ESTIMATES (PER SERVING):
Calories: 280 | Protein: 22g | Carbohydrates: 30g | Fat: 10g | Fiber: 4g

QUICK & EASY TIP: Save time by using pre-made pico de gallo and pre-shredded greens. You can also substitute pre-seasoned frozen fish fillets for an even faster prep.

| 30. | Chipotle Shrimp Tacos |

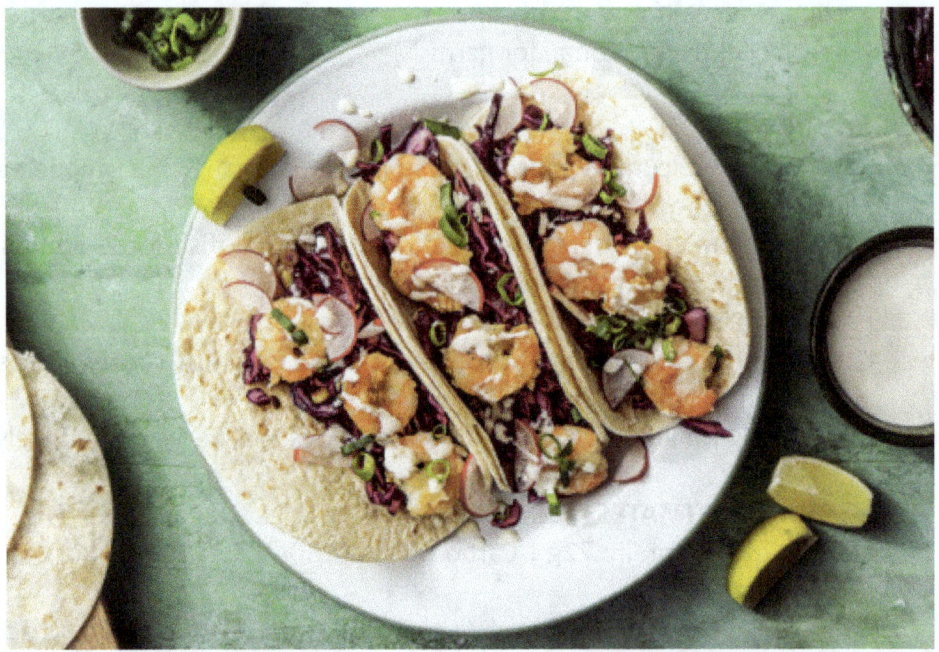

Prep Time: 5 minutes | Cook Time: 8 minutes | Makes: 2

Tacos are a cornerstone of Mexican street food culture, beloved for their versatility and bold flavors. This chipotle shrimp version is inspired by Baja-style seafood tacos from the Pacific coast of Mexico, where fresh shrimp and smoky spices are paired with crisp toppings and zesty crema. It's a perfect weeknight way to bring coastal flavors to your kitchen in minutes.

INGREDIENTS:
- 200g peeled shrimp (medium or large)
- 1 tbsp olive oil
- 1 tsp chipotle powder
- ½ tsp cumin
- Salt and pepper, to taste
- 4 small corn tortillas
- 1 cup shredded cabbage
- ½ avocado, sliced
- 2 tbsp sour cream or Greek yogurt
- 1 tsp lime juice
- Fresh cilantro, for garnish
- Lime wedges, to serve

INSTRUCTIONS:
1. In a bowl, toss shrimp with olive oil, chipotle powder, cumin, salt, and pepper.
2. Heat a skillet over medium-high heat. Add shrimp and cook for 2–3 minutes per side until pink and cooked through.
3. While shrimp cooks, warm tortillas in a dry pan or microwave.
4. Mix sour cream with lime juice to make a quick crema.
5. Assemble tacos: layer cabbage, shrimp, avocado slices, drizzle crema, and top with cilantro.
6. Serve immediately with lime wedges.

NUTRITION ESTIMATES (PER SERVING):
Calories: 380 | Protein: 28g | Carbs: 24g | Fat: 21g | Fiber: 6g

QUICK & EASY TIP: *Add pickled onions or jalapeños for extra punch.*

31. Beef and Black Bean Quesadilla

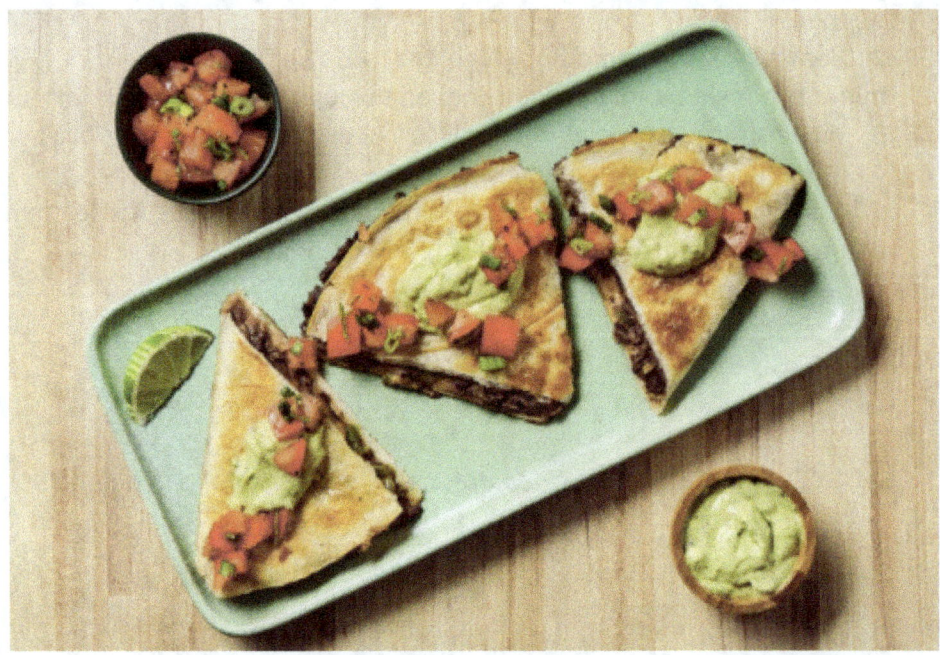

Prep Time: 5 minutes | Cook Time: 10 minutes | Makes: 2

The quesadilla—meaning "little cheesy thing" in Spanish—has long been a Mexican staple, dating back to colonial times. Traditionally made with corn tortillas and local cheese, this modern version uses flour tortillas and adds seasoned beef and beans for a heartier spin. It's a fast, satisfying meal that bridges Mexican tradition with Tex-Mex convenience.

INGREDIENTS:
- 200g ground beef
- ½ cup canned black beans, drained
- ½ small onion, finely chopped
- 1 tsp taco seasoning
- Salt, to taste
- 2 large flour tortillas
- ½ cup shredded cheddar or Mexican cheese blend
- 2 tbsp salsa
- 1 tbsp olive oil
- Optional: sour cream or guacamole for dipping

INSTRUCTIONS:

1. Heat olive oil in a skillet over medium heat. Add onion and cook for 1 minute.
2. Add ground beef, taco seasoning, and a pinch of salt. Cook until browned, about 5–6 minutes.
3. Stir in black beans and cook 1–2 more minutes until heated.
4. Lay tortillas flat. Spread beef mixture on one half, top with cheese and salsa, then fold over.
5. Wipe skillet clean. Toast quesadillas on both sides until golden and crisp, 2–3 minutes per side.
6. Slice and serve with sour cream or guacamole.

NUTRITION ESTIMATES (PER SERVING):
Calories: 450 | Protein: 30g | Carbs: 29g | Fat: 25g | Fiber: 5g

QUICK & EASY TIP: For a spicier kick, add jalapeño slices inside before toasting.

32. Chicken Fajita Skillet

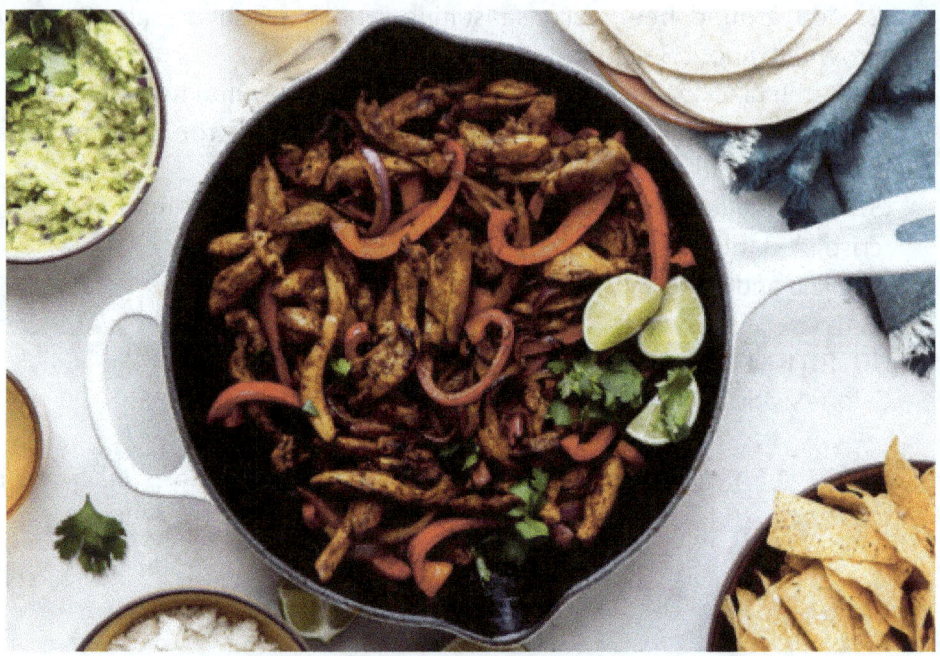

Prep Time: 5 minutes | Cook Time: 10 minutes | Makes: 2

Fajitas originated in Northern Mexico and became popular in Tex-Mex cuisine when Mexican ranch workers grilled skirt steak over open flames. This chicken version skips the grill and goes straight into a skillet — a colorful, sizzling dish with peppers, onions, and bold spices that capture the spirit of a roadside taquería.

INGREDIENTS:
- 200g boneless chicken breast, sliced into strips
- 1 tbsp olive oil
- ½ red bell pepper, sliced
- ½ green bell pepper, sliced
- ½ small red onion, sliced
- 1 tsp fajita seasoning (or mix of paprika, cumin, garlic powder)
- Salt and pepper, to taste
- Juice of ½ lime
- 2 small flour tortillas or lettuce wraps (optional)
- Fresh cilantro and lime wedges, to serve

INSTRUCTIONS:
1. Heat olive oil in a skillet over medium-high heat.

2. Add chicken strips and season with fajita seasoning, salt, and pepper. Cook for 4–5 minutes until browned.
3. Add bell peppers and onion. Cook 3–4 more minutes until vegetables are slightly charred and tender.
4. Squeeze lime juice over the skillet, stir, and remove from heat.
5. Serve hot with tortillas or in lettuce cups, topped with cilantro.

NUTRITION ESTIMATES (PER SERVING):
Calories: 330 | Protein: 34g | Carbs: 14g | Fat: 15g | Fiber: 3g

<u>QUICK & EASY TIP:</u> Use pre-cut chicken and frozen sliced peppers to cut prep time further.

33. Carne Asada Street Tacos

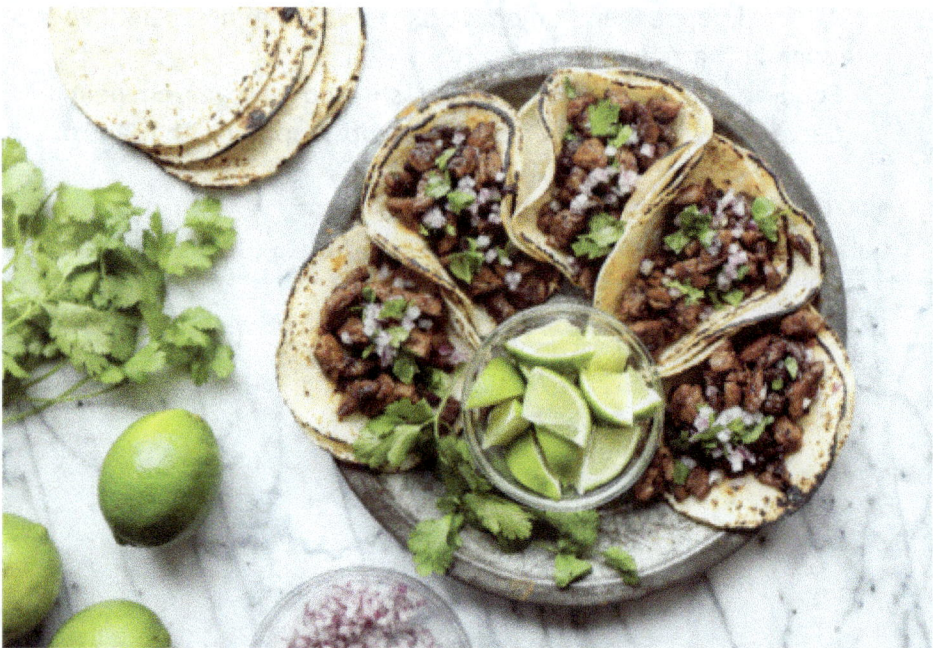

Prep Time: 5 minutes | Cook Time: 8 minutes | Makes: 2

Carne asada, meaning "grilled meat," is a beloved staple in Mexican street food culture. These tacos are quick-pan seared instead of grilled, making them fast and weeknight-friendly — but still full of charred, citrusy flavor.

INGREDIENTS:
- 200g flank or sirloin steak, thinly sliced
- 1 tbsp lime juice
- 1 tbsp olive oil
- ½ tsp ground cumin
- ½ tsp smoked paprika
- Salt and pepper, to taste
- 4 small corn tortillas
- Chopped onion, cilantro, and lime wedges, for topping

INSTRUCTIONS:
1. Toss sliced steak with lime juice, oil, and seasonings.
2. Sear in a hot skillet for 5–6 minutes until browned and cooked through.
3. Warm tortillas.
4. Fill with steak and top with onion, cilantro, and lime juice.

NUTRITION ESTIMATES (PER SERVING):
Calories: 430 | Protein: 34g | Carbs: 22g | Fat: 22g | Fiber: 3g

QUICK & EASY TIP: Use pre-sliced beef or cook in batches to save time. Tortillas can be warmed in the microwave.

34. Chorizo and Potato Skillet

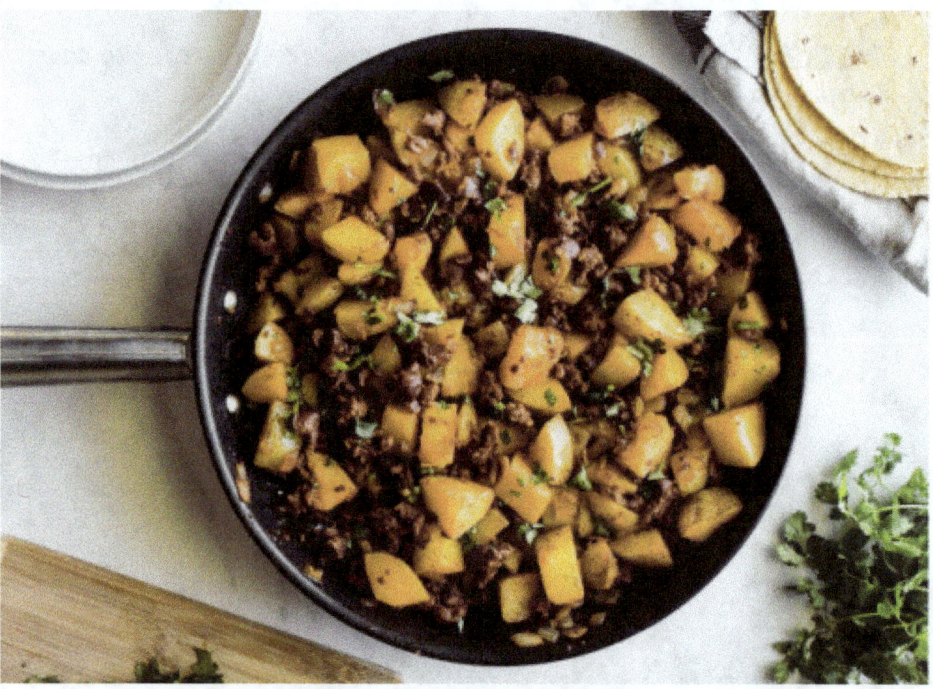

Prep Time: 4 minutes | Cook Time: 10 minutes | Makes: 2

This rustic dish reflects traditional Mexican comfort food, especially in northern and central Mexico. It features spicy chorizo and tender diced potatoes — simple, hearty, and perfect for wrapping in tortillas or enjoying solo.

INGREDIENTS:
- 150g Mexican-style chorizo (casings removed)
- 1 cup cooked or pre-diced potatoes
- ¼ onion, finely chopped
- 1 tbsp oil
- Salt, to taste
- Optional: tortillas, avocado, or hot sauce

INSTRUCTIONS:
1. Heat oil in a skillet. Sauté onion and chorizo for 3–4 minutes.
2. Add potatoes and cook until golden and heated through, about 5–6 minutes.
3. Season and serve as-is or in tortillas.

NUTRITION ESTIMATES (PER SERVING):

Calories: 510 | Protein: 19g | Carbs: 26g | Fat: 36g | Fiber: 3g

QUICK & EASY TIP: Use pre-cooked or leftover potatoes to reduce cook time. Chorizo cooks fast — no need for extra oil if it's fatty.

| 35. | Chicken Tinga Tostadas |

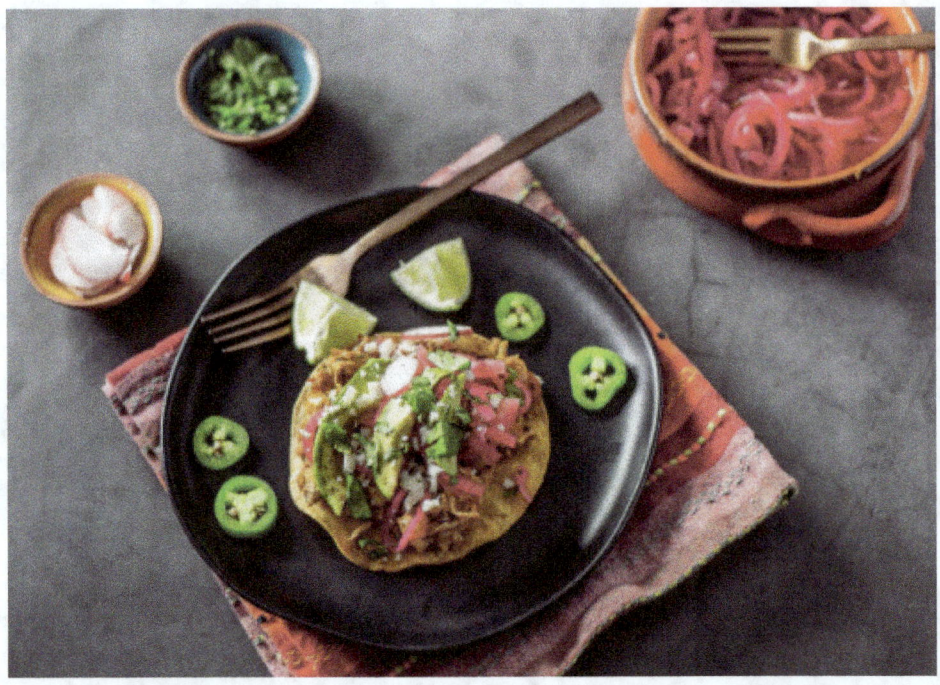

Prep Time: 5 minutes | Cook Time: 10 minutes | Makes: 2

Tinga is a traditional Mexican dish from Puebla, made with shredded chicken in a smoky chipotle-tomato sauce. Served on crispy tostadas, this version is a flavorful, fast dinner with rich depth and a satisfying crunch.

INGREDIENTS:
- 1 cup cooked shredded chicken
- ¼ cup canned crushed tomatoes
- 1 chipotle in adobo, minced
- 2 tbsp chopped onion
- ½ tsp cumin
- 4 tostada shells
- ¼ cup shredded lettuce
- 2 tbsp pickled onions
- 2 tbsp sour cream or crema
- Salt, to taste

INSTRUCTIONS:
1. Sauté onion in a skillet for 2 minutes. Add chipotle, tomatoes, cumin, and chicken. Simmer for 5 minutes.
2. Season with salt.

3. Spoon chicken mixture onto tostadas.
4. Top with lettuce, pickled onions, and a drizzle of sour cream.

NUTRITION ESTIMATES (PER SERVING):
Calories: 440 | Protein: 28g | Carbs: 26g | Fat: 24g | Fiber: 4g

QUICK & EASY TIP: Use rotisserie chicken and pre-made tostada shells to cut down on prep.

| 36. | Veggie Fajita Tacos |

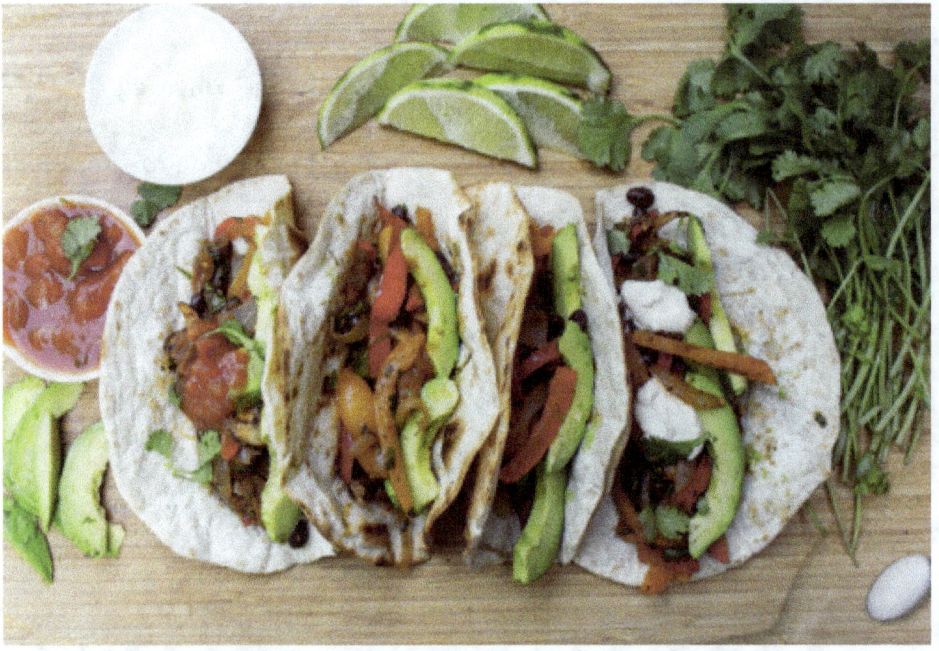

Prep Time: 4 minutes | Cook Time: 10 minutes | Makes: 2

A colorful, plant-forward take on a Mexican classic, veggie fajitas are a go-to in many Mexican households for quick, healthy meals. They sizzle with bell peppers and onions, bringing vibrant texture and smoky flavor.

INGREDIENTS:
- 1 bell pepper, sliced
- ½ red onion, sliced
- 1 small zucchini, sliced
- 1 tbsp olive oil
- ½ tsp chili powder
- ½ tsp cumin
- 4 corn tortillas
- Optional toppings: avocado, salsa, lime

INSTRUCTIONS:
1. Heat oil in a skillet. Sauté vegetables with spices for 6–7 minutes until tender.
2. Warm tortillas.
3. Fill with fajita veggies and top as desired.

NUTRITION ESTIMATES (PER SERVING):

Calories: 350 | Protein: 6g | Carbs: 30g | Fat: 22g | Fiber: 5g

QUICK & EASY TIP: *Pre-slice veggies ahead or buy fajita mixes to speed up prep. Double the batch and refrigerate for later use.*

| 37. | Beef Picadillo Tacos |

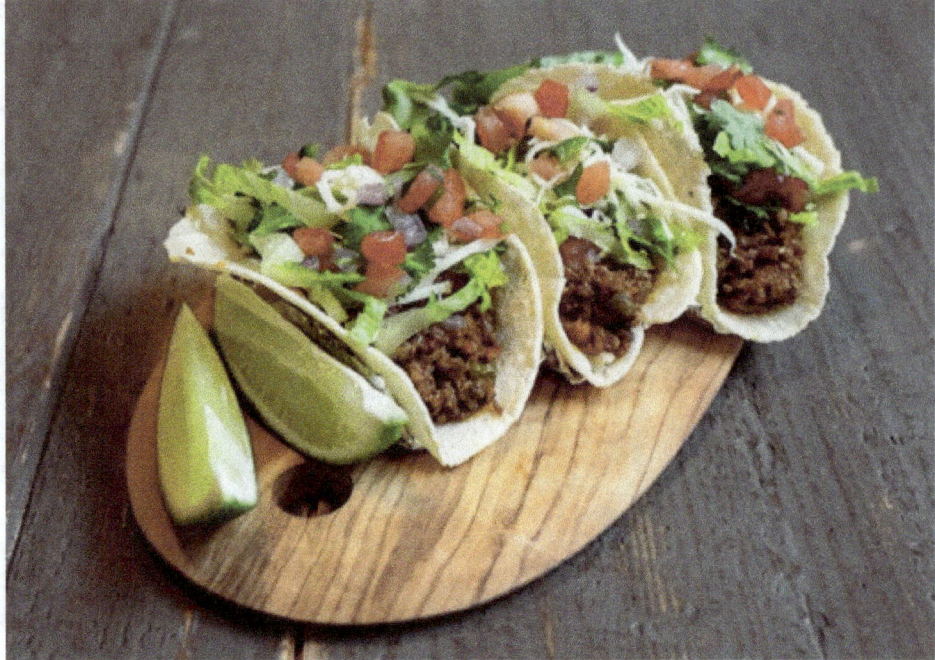

Prep Time: 5 minutes | Cook Time: 9 minutes | Makes: 2

Picadillo, a beloved ground beef dish found throughout Latin America, takes on bold Mexican character with spices, tomatoes, and vegetables. Served in taco form, it's fast, flavorful, and family-friendly.

INGREDIENTS:
- 200g ground beef
- ¼ small onion, diced
- 1 small tomato, diced
- ¼ cup diced potatoes (pre-cooked or frozen)
- 1 tbsp tomato paste
- ½ tsp cumin
- ½ tsp oregano
- Salt and pepper, to taste
- 4 corn tortillas

INSTRUCTIONS:
1. In a skillet, cook ground beef and onion for 3–4 minutes.
2. Add tomato, potatoes, tomato paste, and seasonings. Cook for 5–6 minutes until thickened.
3. Warm tortillas.

4. Spoon beef mixture into tortillas and serve.

NUTRITION ESTIMATES (PER SERVING):
Calories: 460 | Protein: 26g | Carbs: 22g | Fat: 30g | Fiber: 3g

QUICK & EASY TIP: Use pre-cooked or frozen diced potatoes to reduce cooking time. Prepare filling in advance and reheat.

| 38. | Sopa de Lima (Yucatán Lime Soup) |

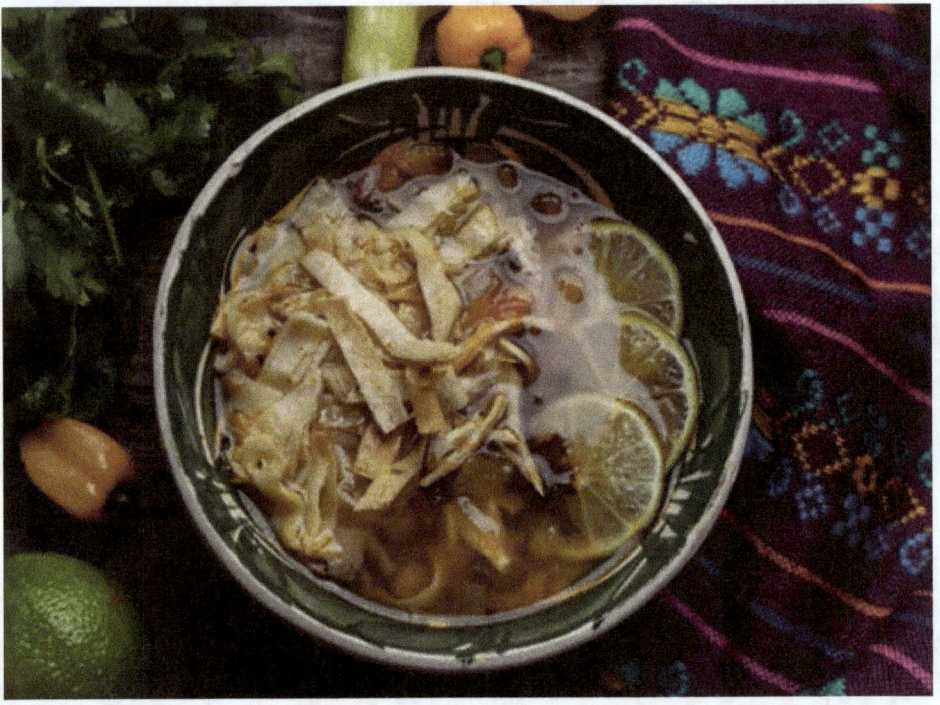

Prep Time: 4 minutes | Cook Time: 10 minutes | Makes: 2

This refreshing chicken soup hails from Mexico's Yucatán Peninsula. It combines zesty lime, tender chicken, and crispy tortilla strips — light, comforting, and surprisingly quick to make with ready ingredients.

INGREDIENTS:
- 1 cup shredded cooked chicken
- 2 cups chicken broth
- ¼ tsp oregano
- ¼ tsp ground cumin
- 2 tbsp lime juice
- Salt, to taste
- 4–6 tortilla strips (toasted or fried)
- Optional: sliced avocado, chopped cilantro

INSTRUCTIONS:
1. Bring broth to a simmer. Add chicken, oregano, cumin, and salt. Cook 5–6 minutes.
2. Stir in lime juice.
3. Ladle into bowls and top with tortilla strips and optional garnishes.

NUTRITION ESTIMATES (PER SERVING):
Calories: 290 | Protein: 26g | Carbs: 8g | Fat: 16g | Fiber: 2g

QUICK & EASY TIP: Use rotisserie chicken and boxed broth to cut prep time. Toast tortilla strips in advance for added crunch.

ITALIAN DINNERS

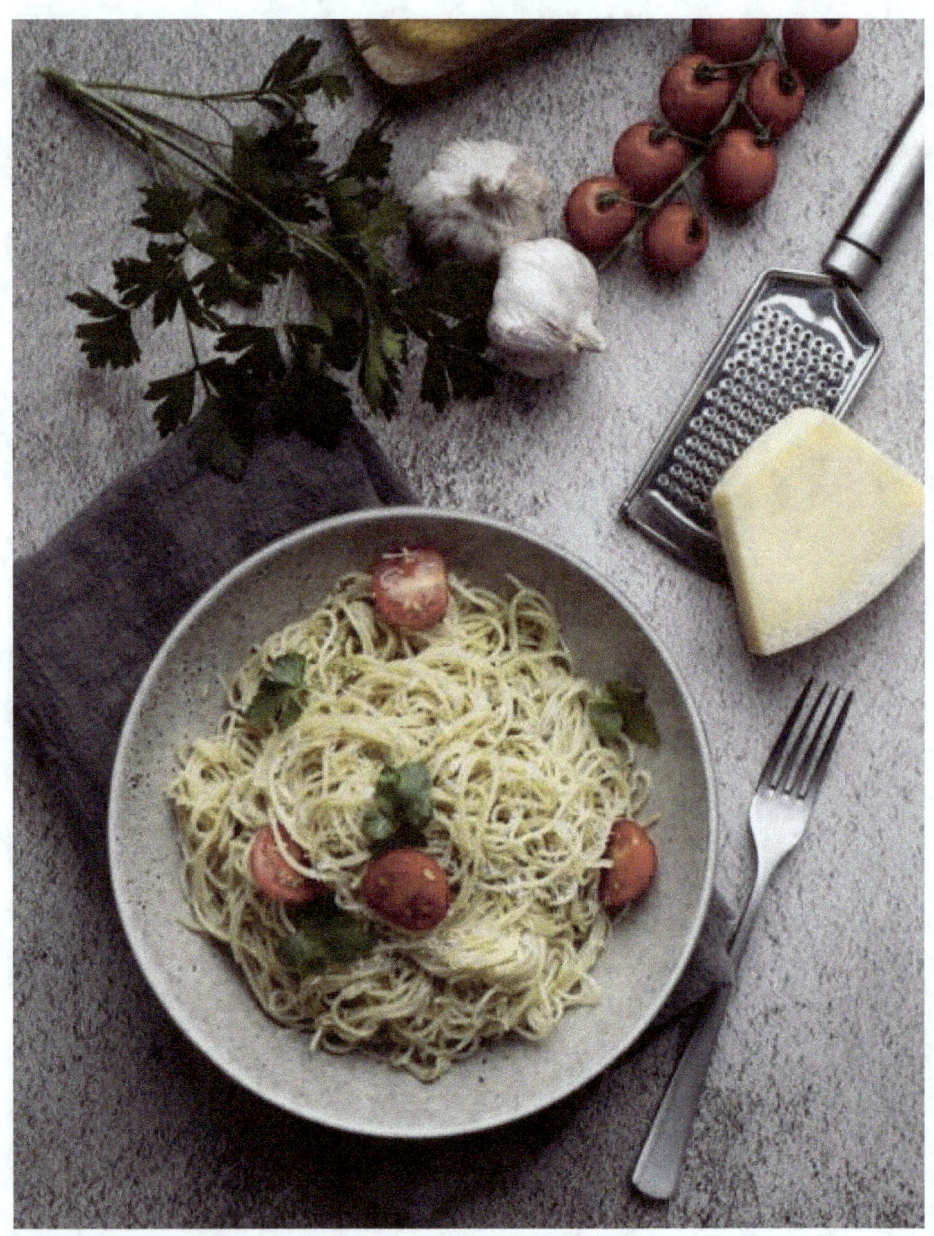

39. Creamy Pesto Gnocchi

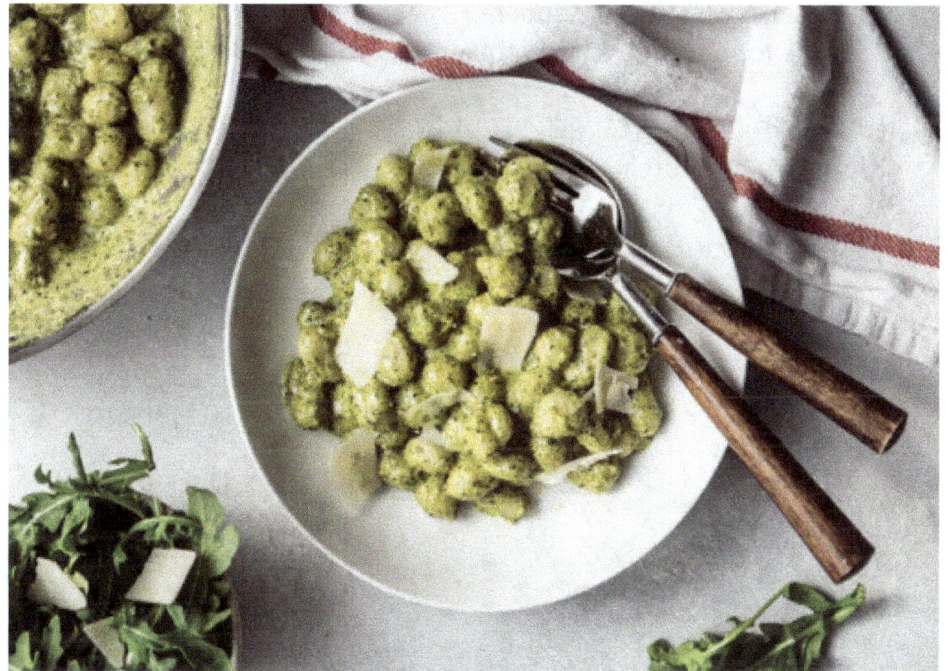

Prep Time: 3 minutes | Cook Time: 10 minutes | Makes: 2

Gnocchi, pillowy dumplings made from potatoes, are a beloved staple of northern Italian kitchens. Traditionally served with butter and sage or tomato sauce, this version uses basil pesto and cream for a quick, comforting dish that feels indulgent yet takes just minutes to make — Italian simplicity at its best.

INGREDIENTS:
- 400g store-bought gnocchi
- 1 tbsp olive oil
- ¼ cup basil pesto
- ¼ cup heavy cream or half-and-half
- 2 tbsp grated Parmesan
- Salt and pepper, to taste
- Fresh basil leaves, for garnish

INSTRUCTIONS:
1. Bring a pot of salted water to a boil. Add gnocchi and cook until they float, about 2–3 minutes. Drain.
2. In a skillet, heat olive oil over medium heat. Add drained gnocchi and lightly sauté for 2 minutes.

3. Stir in pesto and cream. Simmer for 1–2 minutes until the sauce thickens slightly.
4. Season with salt and pepper.
5. Serve topped with Parmesan and fresh basil.

NUTRITION ESTIMATES (PER SERVING):
Calories: 480 | Protein: 10g | Carbs: 55g | Fat: 25g | Fiber: 4g

<u>*QUICK & EASY TIP:*</u> *Swap cream for Greek yogurt for a lighter option.*

40. Caprese Chicken Cutlets

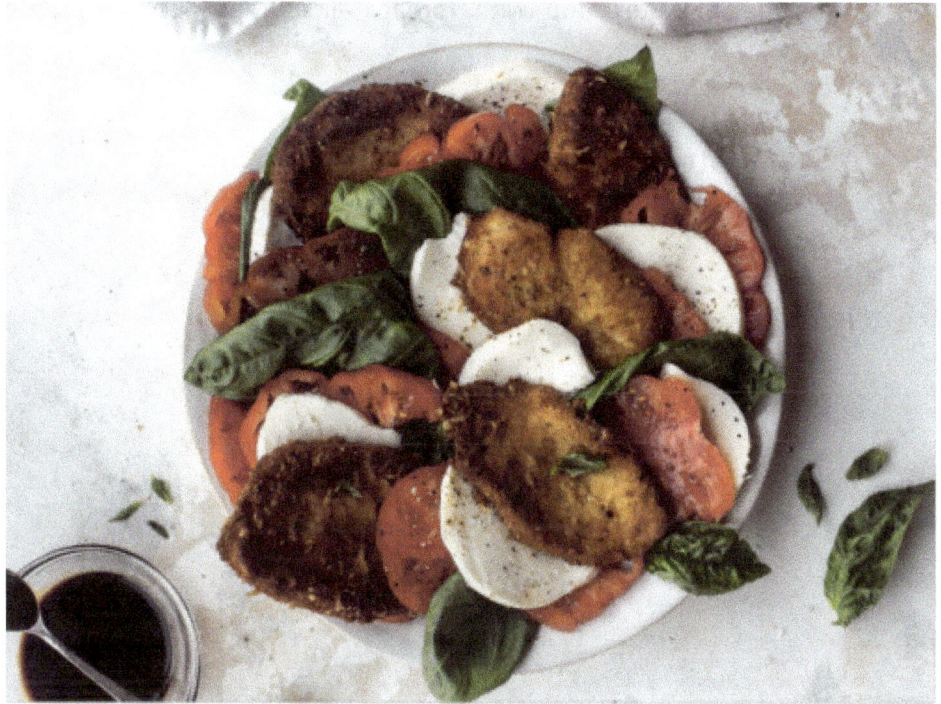

Prep Time: 5 minutes | Cook Time: 10 minutes | Makes: 2

The Caprese salad — fresh mozzarella, tomato, and basil — is a symbol of Italy's culinary elegance. This dish transforms that classic combo into a hot dinner by pairing it with seared chicken cutlets. It's quick, colourful, and captures the Mediterranean spirit in every bite.

INGREDIENTS:
- 2 thin chicken breast cutlets (about 150g each)
- Salt and pepper, to taste
- 1 tbsp olive oil
- 4 slices fresh mozzarella
- 1 medium tomato, sliced
- Fresh basil leaves
- 1 tbsp balsamic glaze or reduction

INSTRUCTIONS:
1. Season chicken with salt and pepper.
2. Heat olive oil in a skillet over medium-high heat. Cook chicken cutlets for 4–5 minutes per side until golden and cooked through.

3. In the last minute of cooking, top each cutlet with mozzarella and cover to melt.
4. Transfer to plates. Top with tomato slices, basil, and a drizzle of balsamic glaze.
5. Serve hot with a side salad or crusty bread.

NUTRITION ESTIMATES (PER SERVING):
Calories: 390 | Protein: 38g | Carbs: 6g | Fat: 23g | Fiber: 1g

QUICK & EASY TIP: For extra flavor, add a sprinkle of dried oregano while cooking the chicken.

41. Garlic Butter Shrimp Spaghetti

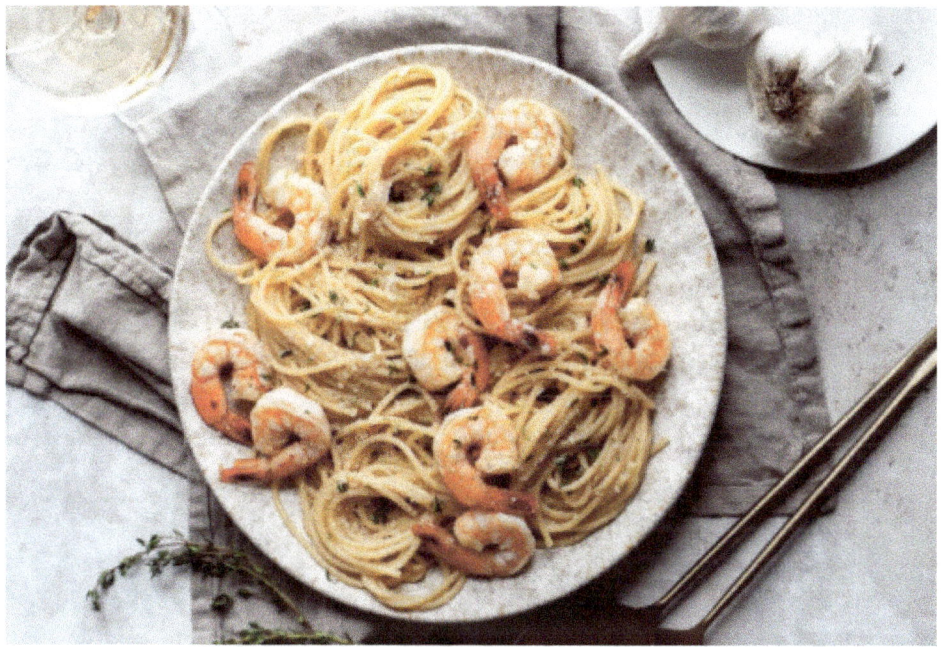

Prep Time: 5 minutes | Cook Time: 10 minutes | Makes: 2

Seafood and pasta are a match made in the southern coastal regions of Italy. This dish echoes the simple elegance of Sicilian cooking — fresh ingredients, quick technique, and a generous use of garlic and olive oil. The garlic butter adds richness, while shrimp brings a touch of briny sweetness, all tied together with al dente spaghetti.

INGREDIENTS:
- 150g spaghetti
- 200g peeled shrimp
- 2 tbsp butter
- 2 tbsp olive oil
- 3 garlic cloves, minced
- Pinch of chili flakes (optional)
- Salt and pepper, to taste
- Juice of ½ lemon
- Fresh parsley, chopped, to garnish
- Grated Parmesan (optional)

INSTRUCTIONS:

1. Cook spaghetti in salted boiling water until al dente, about 8 minutes. Reserve ¼ cup pasta water and drain.
2. Meanwhile, heat butter and olive oil in a skillet over medium heat. Add garlic and chili flakes. Sauté 30 seconds.
3. Add shrimp, season with salt and pepper, and cook 2–3 minutes per side until pink and cooked through.
4. Add drained spaghetti and a splash of pasta water to the skillet. Toss to coat.
5. Finish with lemon juice and parsley. Serve with optional Parmesan.

NUTRITION ESTIMATES (PER SERVING):
Calories: 520 | Protein: 30g | Carbs: 48g | Fat: 24g | Fiber: 2g

**QUICK & EASY TIP:** _Use pre-cooked frozen shrimp to save even more time._

42. Italian Sausage and Pepper Skillet

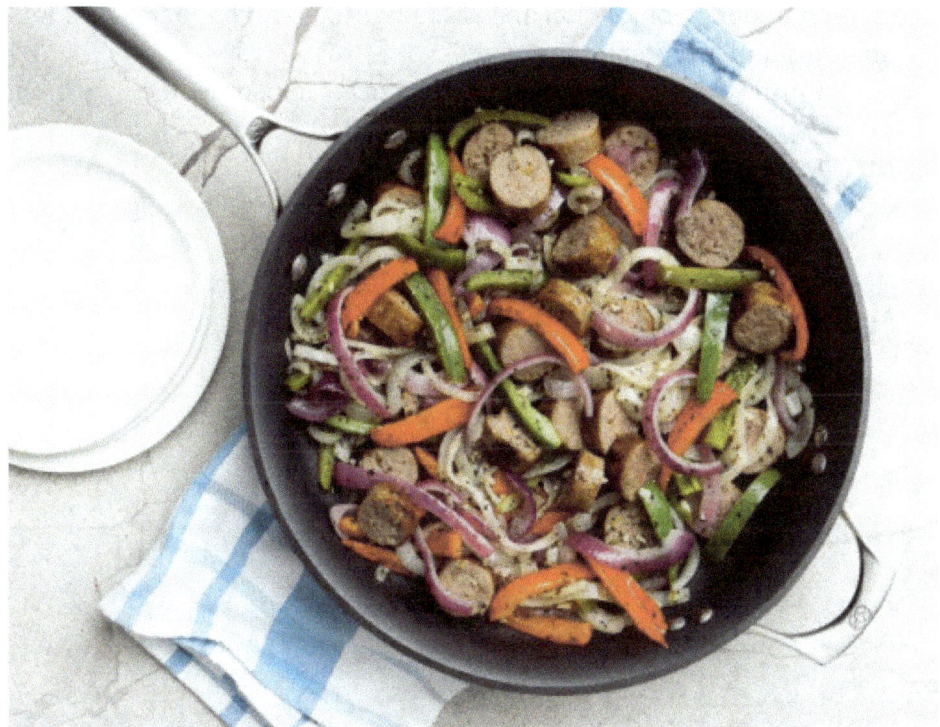

Prep Time: 4 minutes | Cook Time: 10 minutes | Makes: 2

Sausage and peppers is a beloved comfort dish in Italian-American homes, especially in New York and Chicago. Originally brought by Southern Italian immigrants, it combines hearty meat with sweet bell peppers and herbs. This stovetop version skips the long bake and delivers the same rustic flavor in record time.

INGREDIENTS:
- 2 Italian sausages (pork or chicken), sliced
- ½ red bell pepper, sliced
- ½ yellow bell pepper, sliced
- ½ small red onion, sliced
- 1 tbsp olive oil
- ½ tsp Italian seasoning
- Salt and pepper, to taste
- Fresh basil or parsley, to garnish

INSTRUCTIONS:

1. Heat olive oil in a skillet over medium heat. Add sliced sausage and cook 4–5 minutes until browned.
2. Add peppers, onion, Italian seasoning, salt, and pepper. Sauté for 4–5 minutes until vegetables are tender.
3. Garnish with fresh herbs and serve hot — solo, or with crusty bread.

NUTRITION ESTIMATES (PER SERVING):
Calories: 430 | Protein: 22g | Carbs: 12g | Fat: 33g | Fiber: 3g

<u>*QUICK & EASY TIP:*</u> *Use pre-cooked sausage to reduce cooking time further.*

43. Spinach and Ricotta Stuffed Portobellos

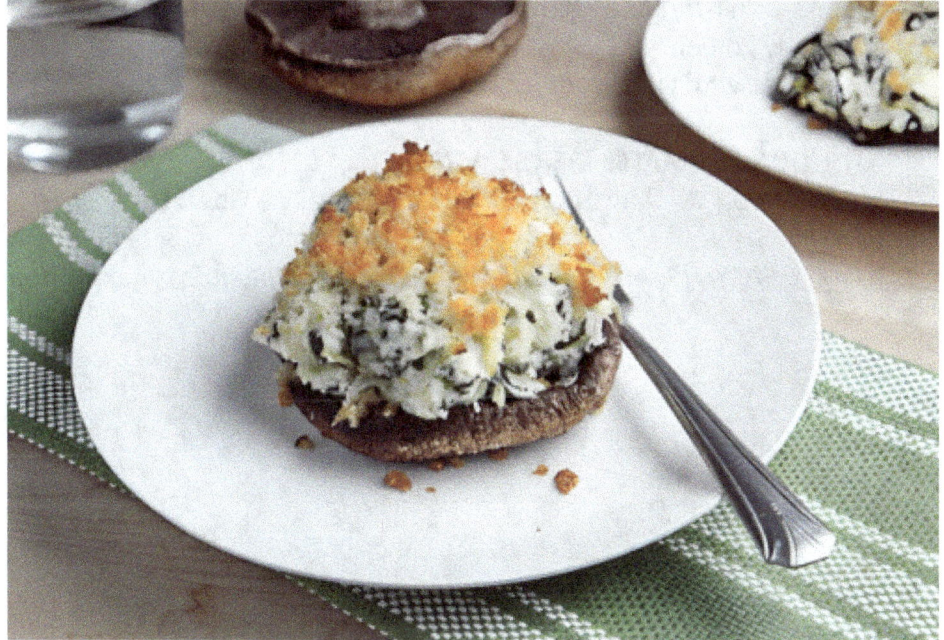

Prep Time: 5 minutes | Cook Time: 10 minutes | Makes: 2

Ricotta and spinach is a classic pairing found in ravioli and cannelloni throughout central Italy. This simplified version skips the pasta but keeps all the creamy, herbaceous flavor by stuffing large portobello mushrooms instead. It's a satisfying vegetarian meal that tastes like comfort, Italian-style.

INGREDIENTS:
- 2 large portobello mushrooms, stems removed
- ½ cup ricotta cheese
- 1 cup baby spinach, chopped
- 2 tbsp grated Parmesan
- 1 garlic clove, minced
- ½ tsp dried oregano
- Salt and pepper, to taste
- 1 tbsp olive oil
- Optional: chili flakes for heat

INSTRUCTIONS:
1. Preheat oven to 200°C (or use an air fryer).
2. In a bowl, mix ricotta, spinach, Parmesan, garlic, oregano, salt, and pepper.

3. Drizzle mushrooms with olive oil and season lightly.
4. Fill each mushroom cap with ricotta mixture.
5. Bake or air-fry for 8–10 minutes until mushrooms are tender and tops are lightly golden.
6. Sprinkle with chili flakes (optional) and serve warm.

NUTRITION ESTIMATES (PER SERVING):
Calories: 310 | Protein: 18g | Carbs: 8g | Fat: 22g | Fiber: 2g

<u>*QUICK & EASY TIP:*</u> *Add sun-dried tomatoes or pine nuts for extra depth.*

| 44. | Prosciutto and Arugula Flatbread |

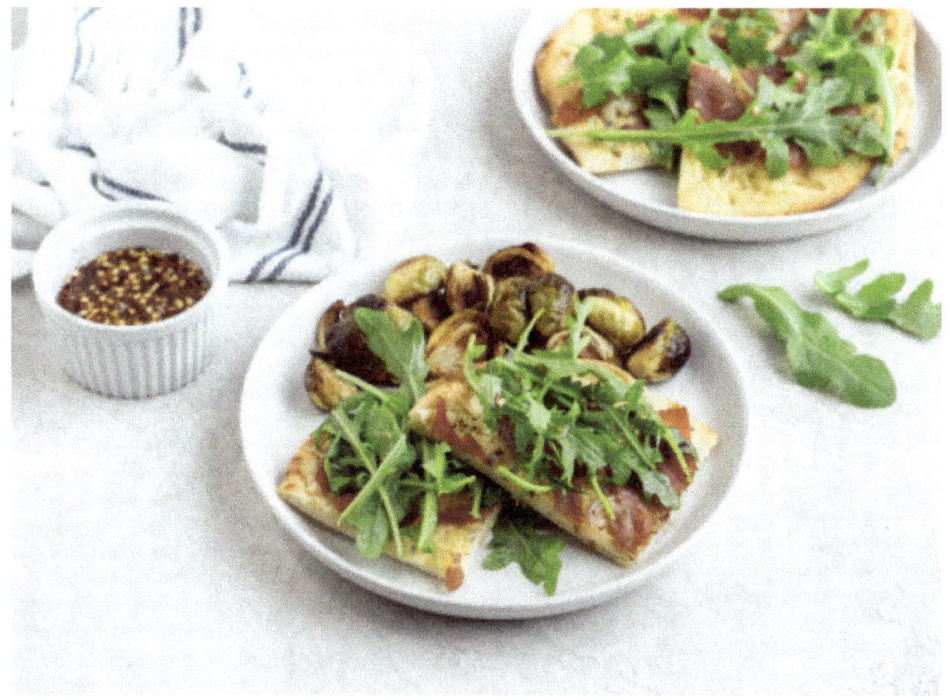

Prep Time: 5 minutes | Cook Time: 8 minutes | Makes: 2

Inspired by the Roman tradition of pizza bianca (white pizza), this flatbread features a thin base topped after baking with cool, peppery arugula and silky prosciutto. It's a popular style in modern Italian aperitivo culture — light, elegant, and ideal for a quick, sophisticated dinner.

INGREDIENTS:
- 1 store-bought flatbread
- 2 tbsp olive oil
- 1 garlic clove, minced
- ½ cup shredded mozzarella or burrata
- 4 slices prosciutto
- 1 cup fresh arugula
- 1 tbsp balsamic glaze
- Salt and cracked black pepper

INSTRUCTIONS:
1. Preheat oven or toaster oven to 200°C.
2. Brush flatbread with olive oil and scatter garlic. Top with cheese.
3. Bake for 6–8 minutes until cheese melts and crust crisps.

4. Remove from oven, then layer with prosciutto and fresh arugula.
5. Drizzle with balsamic glaze and season with salt and pepper. Slice and serve.

NUTRITION ESTIMATES (PER SERVING):
Calories: 420 | Protein: 20g | Carbs: 28g | Fat: 26g | Fiber: 2g

QUICK & EASY TIP: *Swap in smoked salmon or grilled veggies for variation.*

| 45. | Pasta Aglio e Olio |

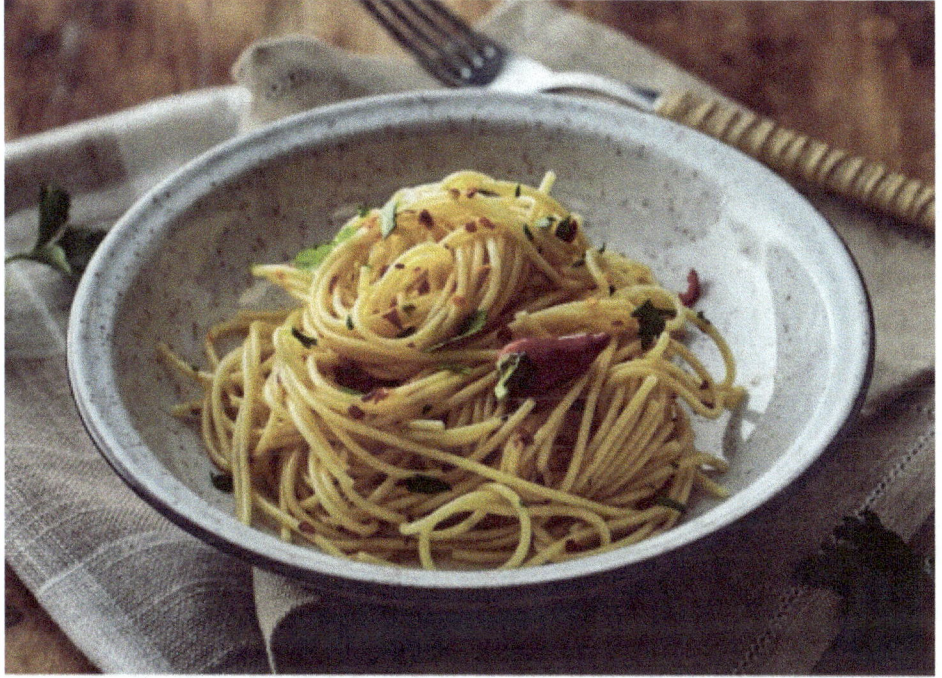

Prep Time: 3 minutes | Cook Time: 10 minutes | Makes: 2

Originating from Naples, Aglio e Olio is one of Italy's simplest and most iconic pasta dishes. It features garlic sautéed in olive oil, finished with parsley and a touch of chili. This minimalist meal showcases how just a few pantry staples can deliver big flavor.

INGREDIENTS:
- 160g spaghetti or linguine
- 3 tbsp olive oil
- 3 garlic cloves, thinly sliced
- ¼ tsp chili flakes
- Salt, to taste
- 2 tbsp chopped fresh parsley
- Grated Parmesan (optional)

INSTRUCTIONS:
1. Boil pasta in salted water until al dente. Reserve ¼ cup pasta water.
2. Sauté garlic in olive oil over medium heat for 1–2 minutes until golden.
3. Add chili flakes and reserved pasta water.
4. Toss drained pasta into the pan and mix well.

5. Garnish with parsley and Parmesan if using.

NUTRITION ESTIMATES (PER SERVING):
Calories: 480 | Protein: 12g | Carbs: 58g | Fat: 22g | Fiber: 3g

QUICK & EASY TIP: *Use pre-minced garlic and boil pasta while prepping sauce to save time.*

46.	Chicken Piccata

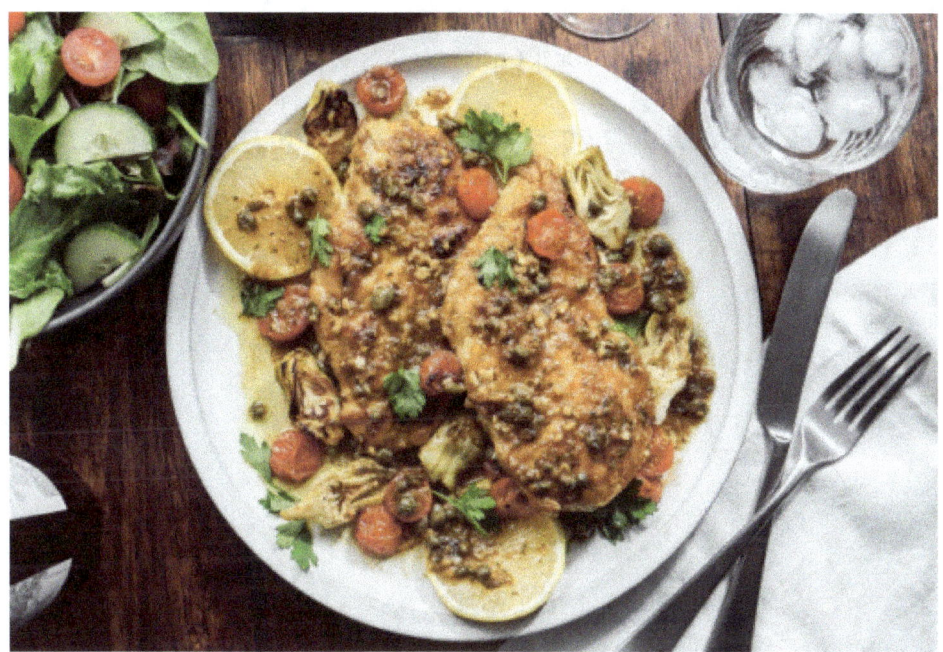

Prep Time: 5 minutes | Cook Time: 9 minutes | Makes: 2

Chicken Piccata is a classic dish from Southern Italy, featuring lightly pan-fried chicken in a tangy lemon-caper butter sauce. It's elegant enough for guests, yet simple and fast enough for weeknight dinners.

INGREDIENTS:
- 2 boneless, thin chicken breast cutlets
- 2 tbsp flour
- 1 tbsp olive oil
- 1 tbsp butter
- ¼ cup chicken broth
- 1 tbsp lemon juice
- 1 tbsp capers
- ½ cup cherry tomatoes, roasted
- Chopped parsley, to garnish

INSTRUCTIONS:
1. Lightly coat chicken with flour.
2. Heat oil and butter in a pan. Cook chicken for 3–4 minutes per side until golden and cooked through.
3. Add broth, lemon juice, and capers. Simmer 2–3 minutes.
4. Stir in roasted tomatoes and cook for 1 minute until warmed through.

5. Spoon sauce and tomatoes over chicken and garnish with parsley.

NUTRITION ESTIMATES (PER SERVING):
Calories: 360 | Protein: 30g | Carbs: 7g | Fat: 23g | Fiber: 1g

QUICK & EASY TIP: *Use pre-sliced chicken or cutlets to speed up cooking. Sauce can be pre-mixed and stored cold.*

47. Margherita Skillet Pizza

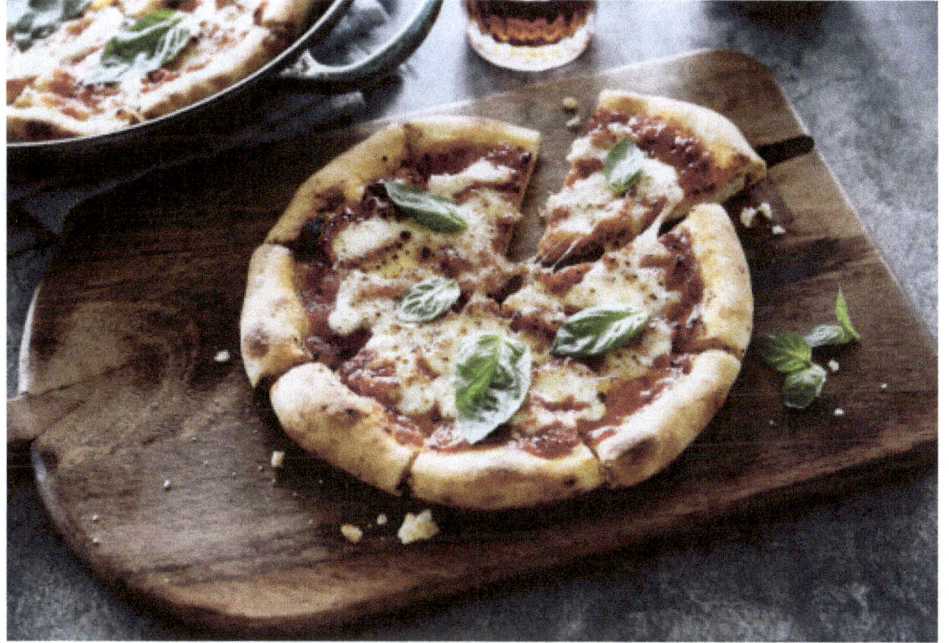

Prep Time: 4 minutes | Cook Time: 10 minutes | Makes: 2

Named after Queen Margherita of Savoy, this iconic pizza mirrors the colors of the Italian flag — red tomatoes, white mozzarella, and green basil. This stovetop version skips the oven for a lightning-fast dinner.

INGREDIENTS:
- 1 small pre-made pizza crust or naan
- ⅓ cup crushed tomatoes
- 1 tsp olive oil
- ½ tsp dried oregano
- ½ cup fresh mozzarella, sliced
- Fresh basil leaves
- Salt and pepper, to taste

INSTRUCTIONS:
1. Heat a skillet over medium heat.
2. Brush crust with olive oil. Spread tomatoes and sprinkle oregano.
3. Add mozzarella and season.
4. Cover and cook in skillet for 6–7 minutes until cheese melts and bottom is crisp.
5. Garnish with basil and serve.

NUTRITION ESTIMATES (PER SERVING):
Calories: 420 | Protein: 17g | Carbs: 36g | Fat: 24g | Fiber: 3g

<u>*QUICK & EASY TIP:*</u> *Use pre-sliced cheese and crusts. No oven needed — just a covered skillet.*

| 48. | Tuna Puttanesca |

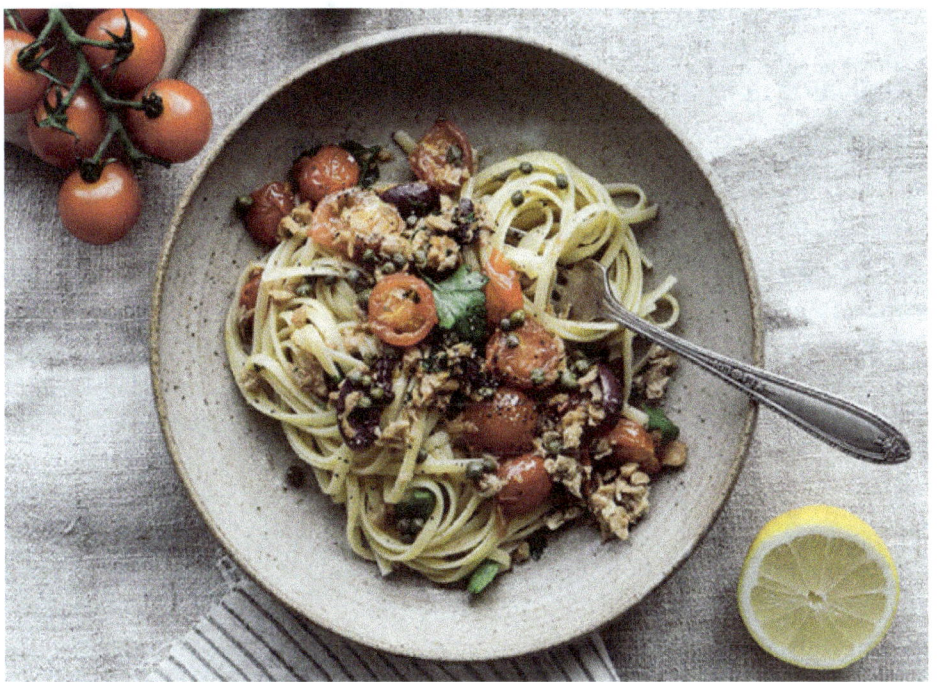

Prep Time: 4 minutes | Cook Time: 10 minutes | Makes: 2

Originating from Naples, Pasta alla Puttanesca is bold and briny, featuring olives, capers, and garlic. Adding canned tuna turns it into a protein-packed meal, making it a pantry-based Italian dinner favorite.

INGREDIENTS:
- 160g spaghetti
- 1 tbsp olive oil
- 2 garlic cloves, minced
- 4–5 olives, sliced
- 1 tbsp capers
- 1 small can tuna in olive oil, drained
- ½ cup crushed tomatoes
- Salt and pepper, to taste

INSTRUCTIONS:
1. Cook pasta in salted water.
2. While pasta cooks, sauté garlic in olive oil for 1 minute.
3. Add olives, capers, tomatoes, and tuna. Simmer 5 minutes.
4. Toss with drained pasta and serve.

NUTRITION ESTIMATES (PER SERVING):
Calories: 470 | Protein: 28g | Carbs: 45g | Fat: 20g | Fiber: 3g

<u>*QUICK & EASY TIP:*</u> *Use canned tuna and jarred olives/capers to minimize prep. Start sauce as pasta boils.*

49. Chicken Marsala Skillet

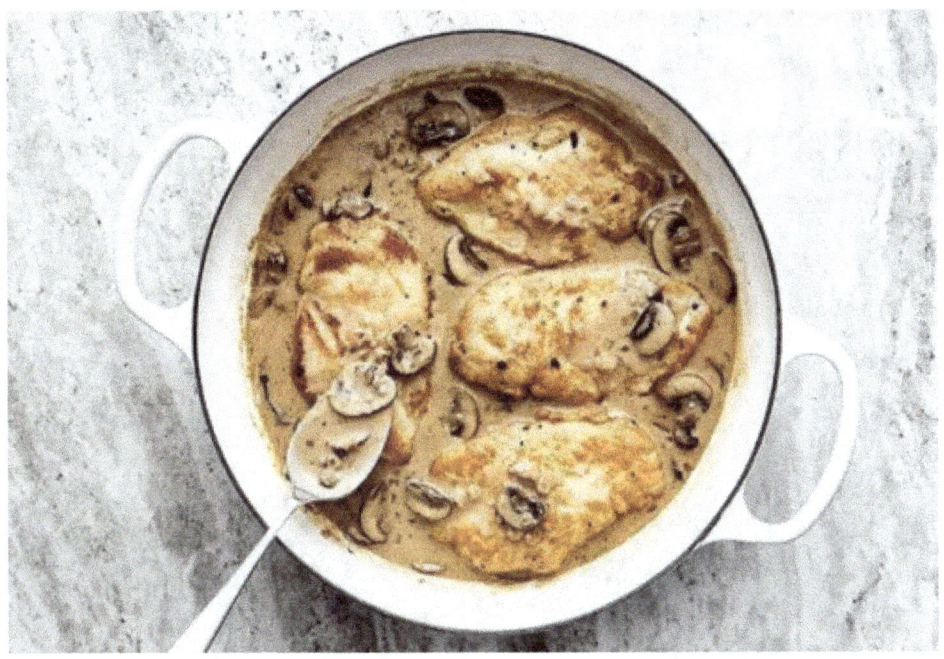

Prep Time: 4 minutes | Cook Time: 10 minutes | Makes: 2

A Northern Italian favorite, Chicken Marsala features tender chicken breast in a rich mushroom and Marsala wine sauce. Its roots trace back to Sicily, where Marsala wine originates, but the dish became a restaurant staple across Italy and the U.S.

INGREDIENTS:
- 2 thin chicken breast cutlets
- 2 tbsp flour
- 1 tbsp olive oil
- 1 tbsp butter
- ½ cup mushrooms, sliced
- ¼ cup Marsala wine
- Salt and pepper, to taste
- Chopped parsley (for garnish)

INSTRUCTIONS:
1. Lightly dredge chicken in flour.
2. Heat oil and butter in a skillet. Cook chicken 3–4 minutes per side.
3. Add mushrooms and sauté for 2 minutes.
4. Pour in Marsala wine and simmer 2–3 minutes.
5. Serve with sauce and garnish with parsley.

NUTRITION ESTIMATES (PER SERVING):
Calories: 390 | Protein: 32g | Carbs: 10g | Fat: 23g | Fiber: 1g

QUICK & EASY TIP: *Use pre-sliced mushrooms and chicken cutlets to minimize prep. Sauce reduces quickly due to wine's low moisture content.*

50. White Bean and Kale Sauté

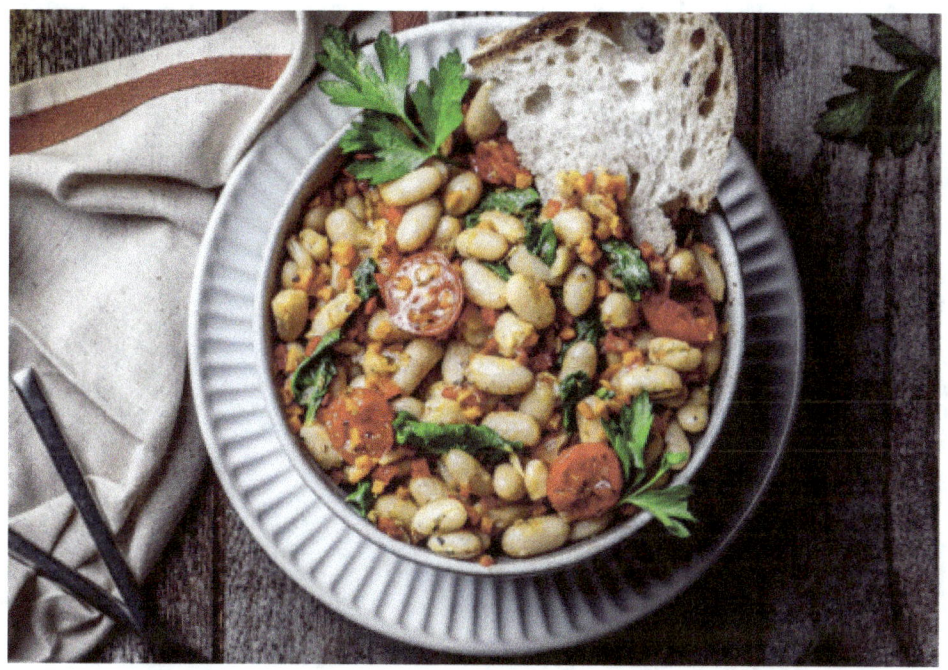

Prep Time: 3 minutes | Cook Time: 9 minutes | Makes: 2

This rustic Tuscan-inspired dish brings together white beans, leafy greens, garlic, and olive oil in a quick, protein-rich vegetarian dinner. It's hearty, humble, and full of flavor with pantry staples.

INGREDIENTS:
- 1 tbsp olive oil
- 2 garlic cloves, minced
- 1 cup canned cannellini beans, drained
- 1 cup chopped kale
- ¼ tsp chili flakes
- Salt and pepper, to taste
- Grated Parmesan (optional)

INSTRUCTIONS:
1. Heat olive oil in a skillet. Sauté garlic for 1 minute.
2. Add kale and cook for 2–3 minutes until wilted.
3. Add beans, chili flakes, salt, and pepper. Cook for 4–5 minutes.
4. Top with Parmesan if desired.

NUTRITION ESTIMATES (PER SERVING):
Calories: 290 | Protein: 12g | Carbs: 22g | Fat: 18g | Fiber: 6g

QUICK & EASY TIP: *Use pre-washed kale and canned beans for ultra-quick prep. Great with toasted bread or as-is.*

INDIAN DINNERS

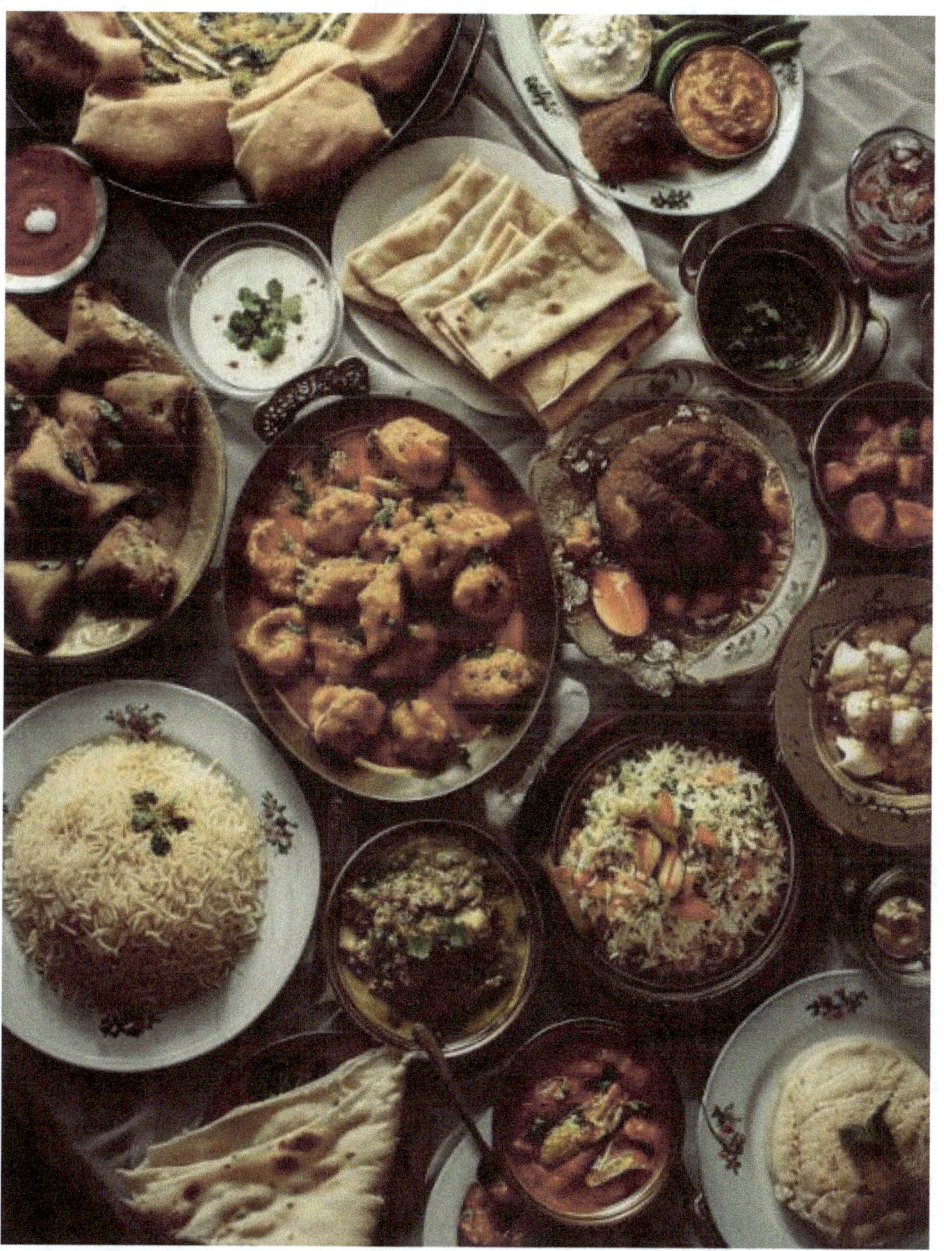

51. Egg Curry (Anda Curry)

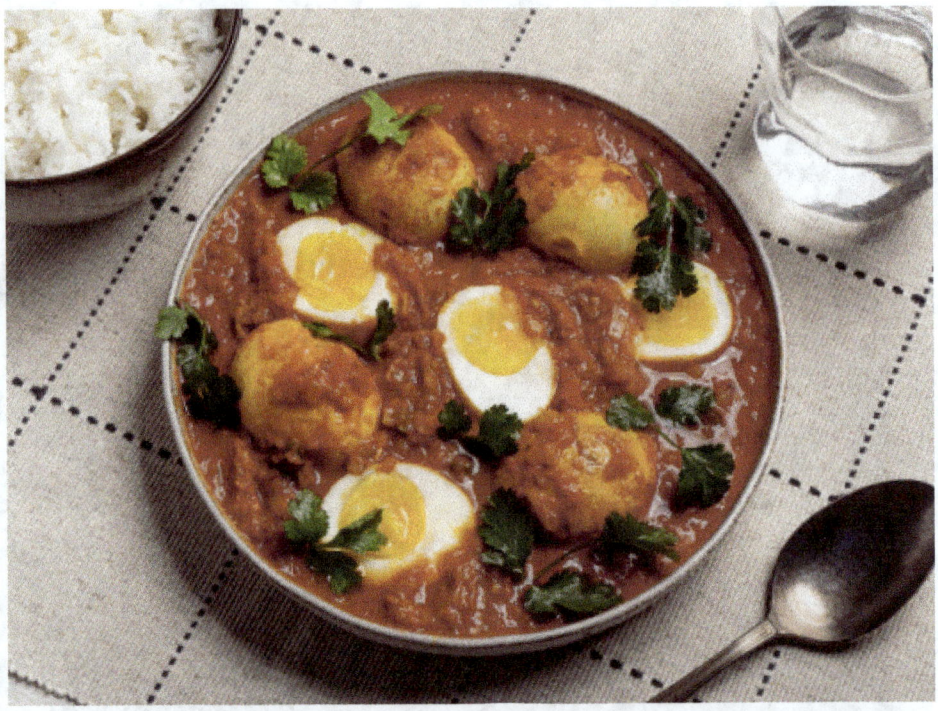

Prep Time: 5 minutes | Cook Time: 10 minutes | Makes: 2

Egg curry is a beloved staple in many Indian homes — especially in Bengal, Punjab, and Kerala — where it's served as a hearty, everyday meal. This quick version skips slow simmering but retains all the warmth and spice, perfect for a speedy dinner with rice or parathas.

INGREDIENTS:
- 4 hard-boiled eggs, peeled
- 1 tbsp oil
- ½ tsp cumin seeds
- ½ onion, finely chopped
- 1 tomato, finely chopped
- 1 garlic clove, minced
- ½ tsp turmeric
- ½ tsp chili powder
- ½ tsp coriander powder
- ¼ tsp garam masala
- Salt, to taste
- ½ cup water
- Fresh coriander, for garnish

INSTRUCTIONS:
1. Heat oil in a pan over medium heat. Add cumin seeds and let them sizzle.
2. Add onion and garlic, sauté for 2–3 minutes. Add tomato, turmeric, chili, coriander powder, and salt. Cook until tomatoes soften, about 3 minutes.
3. Add water and bring to a simmer.
4. Gently add boiled eggs and cook for 3–4 minutes, turning to coat in masala.
5. Sprinkle garam masala and garnish with fresh coriander. Serve hot with rice or chapati.

NUTRITION ESTIMATES (PER SERVING):
Calories: 310 | Protein: 18g | Carbs: 9g | Fat: 22g | Fiber: 2g

QUICK & EASY TIP: Slice eggs before adding for more flavor absorption.

52. Jeera Rice with Tadka Dal

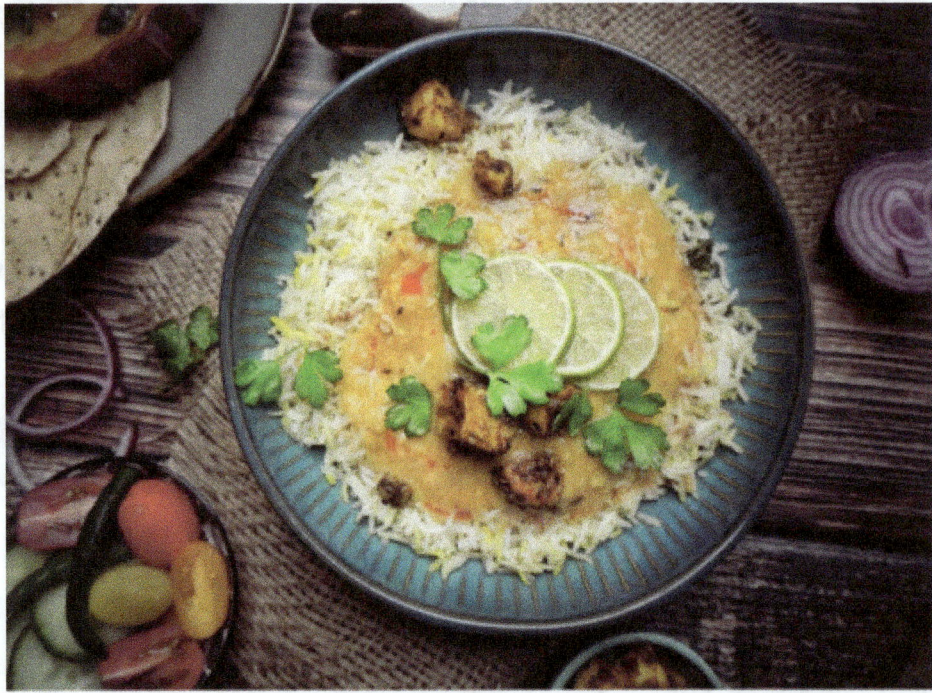

Prep Time: 5 minutes | Cook Time: 10 minutes | Makes: 2

Jeera rice and dal is a classic North Indian comfort dinner, simple yet rich in flavor. "Tadka" means tempered spices — a technique that brings life to plain lentils with sizzling cumin, garlic, and chili in hot oil. Combined with fragrant cumin rice, it's a soulful, everyday meal ready in minutes.

INGREDIENTS:
FOR JEERA RICE:
- 1 cup cooked basmati rice (or microwaveable packet)
- 1 tsp ghee or oil
- ½ tsp cumin seeds
- Salt, to taste

FOR TADKA DAL:
- 1 cup cooked yellow moong dal (or canned lentils)
- 1 tbsp ghee or oil
- 1 garlic clove, sliced
- 1 dried red chili or pinch chili flakes
- ½ tsp cumin seeds
- ¼ tsp turmeric
- Salt, to taste
- Fresh coriander, for garnish

INSTRUCTIONS:
1. Heat ghee in a small pan for the rice. Add cumin seeds, let sizzle, then toss in the rice and salt. Stir-fry 2–3 minutes. Set aside.
2. In another pan, heat ghee for the dal. Add cumin seeds, garlic, and chili. Sauté until garlic is golden.
3. Add turmeric and cooked dal. Simmer 3–4 minutes, adjust salt, and finish with coriander.
4. Serve hot with jeera rice.

NUTRITION ESTIMATES (PER SERVING):
Calories: 420 | Protein: 14g | Carbs: 46g | Fat: 18g | Fiber: 7g

QUICK & EASY TIP: *Add spinach or tomato to dal for variation.*

53. Spinach and Paneer Curry

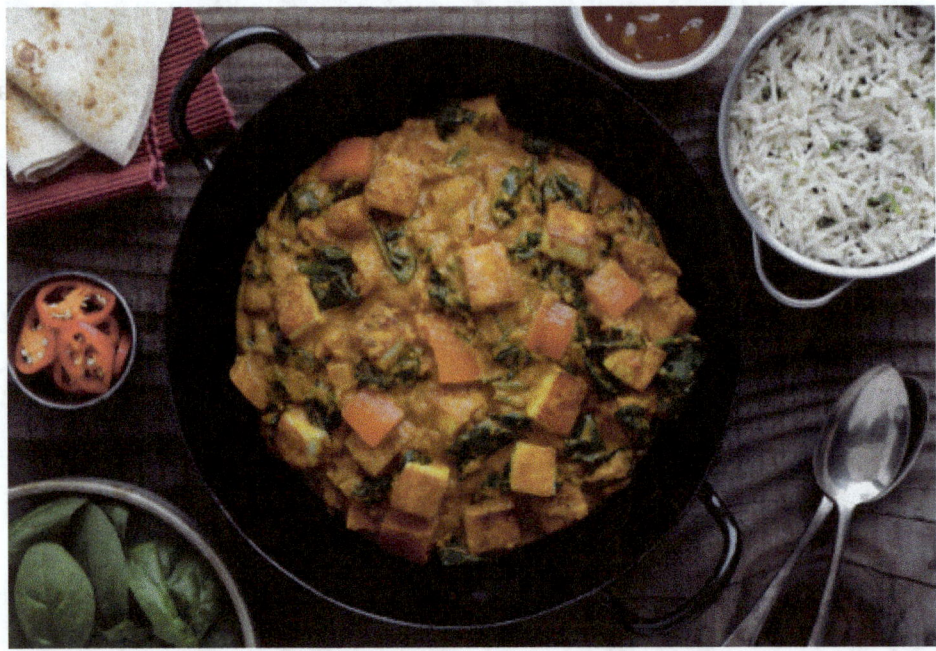

Prep Time: 5 minutes | Cook Time: 10 minutes | Makes: 2

Palak Paneer is a North Indian classic made by simmering paneer cubes in a creamy spinach gravy. Traditionally made slowly, this shortcut version uses blanched or frozen spinach and a quick blend to achieve authentic taste in minutes — all the goodness of greens with indulgent paneer.

INGREDIENTS:
- 200g paneer, cubed
- 1 tbsp oil or ghee
- 1 garlic clove, minced
- 1 green chili, optional
- 2 cups spinach leaves (blanched) or 1 cup frozen spinach
- ¼ cup water
- ½ tsp cumin seeds
- ¼ tsp turmeric
- ½ tsp garam masala
- Salt, to taste
- 1 tbsp cream or yogurt (optional)
- Roti or rice, to serve

INSTRUCTIONS:
1. Blend spinach, green chili, and water into a smooth purée.

2. In a skillet, heat oil and add cumin seeds. Add garlic and sauté 30 seconds.
3. Add turmeric, salt, and spinach purée. Simmer for 2–3 minutes.
4. Stir in paneer and garam masala. Simmer 3–4 more minutes. Add cream if using.
5. Serve hot with roti or jeera rice.

NUTRITION ESTIMATES (PER SERVING):
Calories: 410 | Protein: 19g | Carbs: 12g | Fat: 32g | Fiber: 4g

QUICK & EASY TIP: For extra depth, stir in 1 tsp dried fenugreek (kasuri methi) before serving.

54. Quick Chicken Korma

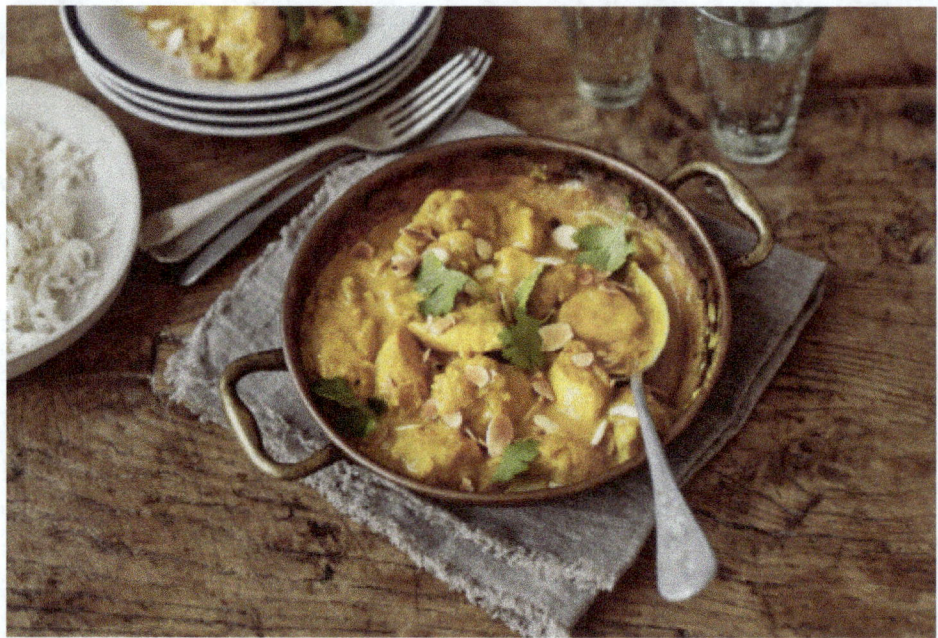

Prep Time: 5 minutes | Cook Time: 9 minutes | Makes: 2

Chicken Korma is a creamy, mildly spiced Mughlai dish known for its rich texture and aromatic flavors. Traditionally slow-cooked, this shortcut version retains the essence of korma using pantry staples and boneless chicken for a fast, satisfying dinner.

INGREDIENTS:
- 250g boneless chicken, cut into small pieces
- 2 tbsp yogurt
- 1 small onion, finely chopped
- 1 tbsp oil or ghee
- 1 tsp ginger-garlic paste
- ¼ tsp turmeric
- ½ tsp coriander powder
- ¼ tsp garam masala
- ¼ tsp chili powder
- Salt, to taste
- 2 tbsp cream or coconut milk (optional)
- 2 tbsp chopped cilantro

INSTRUCTIONS:

1. Heat oil in a pan. Sauté onions for 2–3 minutes until golden.
2. Add ginger-garlic paste. Cook for 30 seconds.
3. Add chicken, yogurt, turmeric, coriander, chili powder, and salt. Mix well.
4. Cover and cook on medium for 5–6 minutes until chicken is tender.
5. Stir in cream (if using) and garam masala. Simmer for 1 minute.
6. Garnish with cilantro and serve with rice or naan.

NUTRITION ESTIMATES (PER SERVING):
Calories: 390 | Protein: 30g | Carbs: 8g | Fat: 26g | Fiber: 1g

QUICK & EASY TIP: Use pre-chopped chicken and a nonstick pan for quick cooking. Yogurt tenderizes quickly, so no marination needed.

55. Achari Chicken (Pickled-Spiced Chicken)

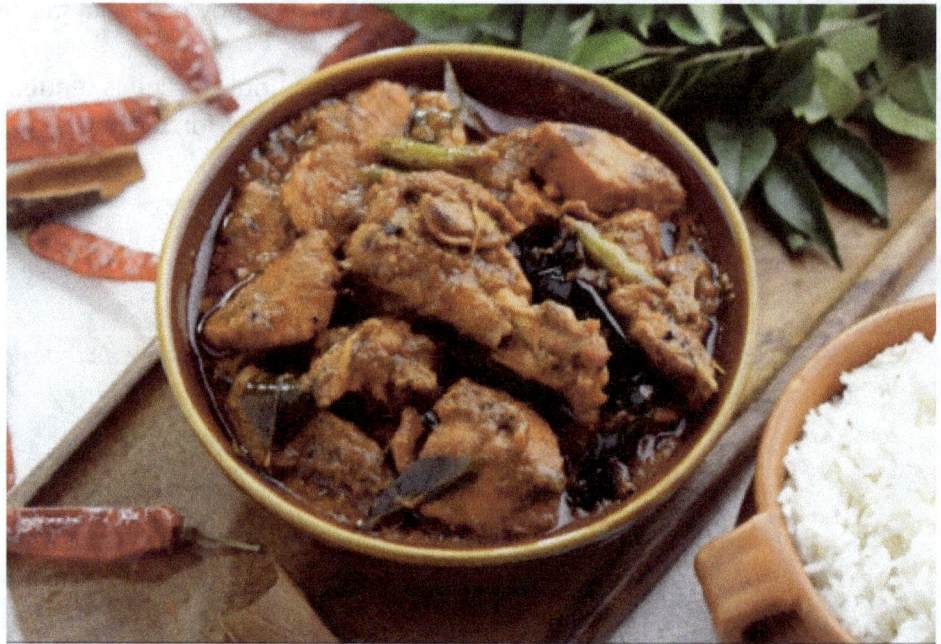

Prep Time: 4 minutes | Cook Time: 10 minutes | Makes: 2

Achari Chicken is a spicy North Indian dish inspired by the bold, tangy flavors of Indian pickles (achar). This express version brings out that signature punch in under 15 minutes, using minimal ingredients and no grinding of spices.

INGREDIENTS:
- 250g boneless chicken, thinly sliced
- 1 tbsp mustard oil or vegetable oil
- 1 tsp ginger-garlic paste
- ½ tsp nigella seeds (kalonji)
- ½ tsp fennel seeds
- ¼ tsp mustard seeds
- ½ tsp chili powder
- ¼ tsp turmeric
- ½ tsp cumin powder
- Salt, to taste
- 1 tbsp yogurt
- 1 tsp lemon juice

INSTRUCTIONS:

1. Heat oil in a pan. Add mustard seeds, nigella seeds, and fennel seeds. Let them splutter.
2. Add ginger-garlic paste. Sauté for 30 seconds.
3. Add chicken, turmeric, chili powder, cumin, and salt. Sauté 5–6 minutes.
4. Add yogurt and stir well. Cook for 2 more minutes until chicken is fully done.
5. Drizzle lemon juice. Mix and serve hot.

NUTRITION ESTIMATES (PER SERVING):
Calories: 360 | Protein: 32g | Carbs: 6g | Fat: 22g | Fiber: 2g

QUICK & EASY TIP: Slice chicken thinly for faster cooking. Spice mix can be pre-made in batches for repeat use.

56. Mixed Vegetable Curry

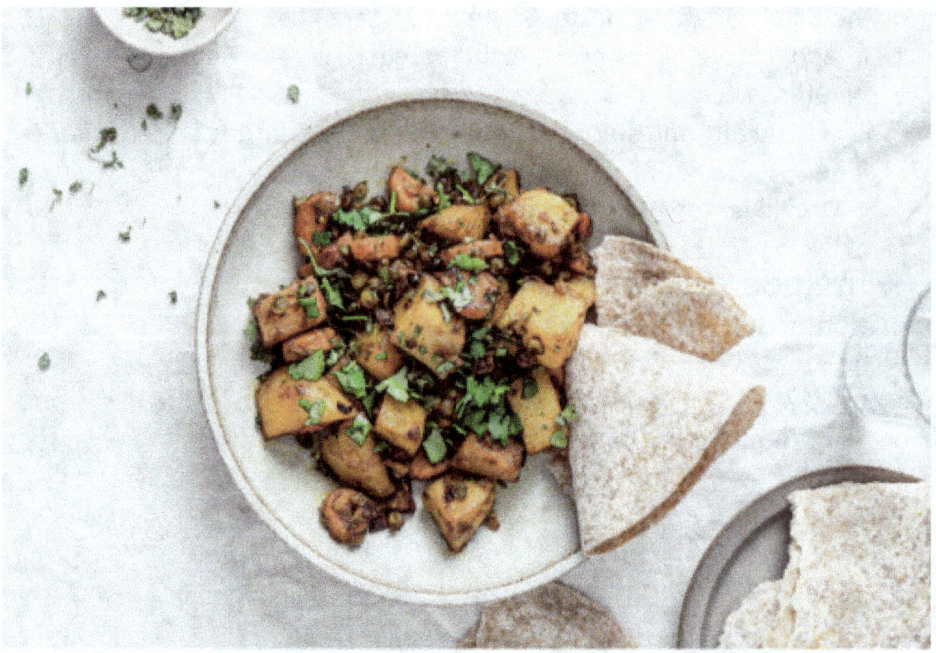

Prep Time: 4 minutes | Cook Time: 10 minutes | Makes: 2

Mixed Vegetable Curry is a beloved Indian household dish that adapts to whatever vegetables you have on hand. This speedy version uses a light onion-tomato base and cooks quickly using frozen or pre-chopped vegetables.

INGREDIENTS:
- 2 cups mixed vegetables (carrot, peas, green beans, potatoes—fresh or frozen)
- 1 tbsp oil
- 1 small onion, finely chopped
- 1 tomato, chopped
- 1 tsp ginger-garlic paste
- ½ tsp turmeric
- ½ tsp coriander powder
- ½ tsp garam masala
- ½ tsp chili powder
- Salt, to taste
- ½ cup water
- Chopped cilantro for garnish

INSTRUCTIONS:

1. Heat oil. Sauté onions for 2 minutes until soft.
2. Add ginger-garlic paste and cook for 30 seconds.
3. Stir in tomatoes and spices. Cook until tomatoes soften.
4. Add vegetables, salt, and water. Cover and cook for 5–7 minutes until veggies are tender.
5. Finish with garam masala and garnish with cilantro.

NUTRITION ESTIMATES (PER SERVING):
Calories: 190 | Protein: 5g | Carbs: 28g | Fat: 7g | Fiber: 6g

QUICK & EASY TIP: Use pre-cut or frozen mixed vegetables to save prep time. Cook uncovered at the end to reduce water for a thicker curry.

57. Chicken Jalfrezi

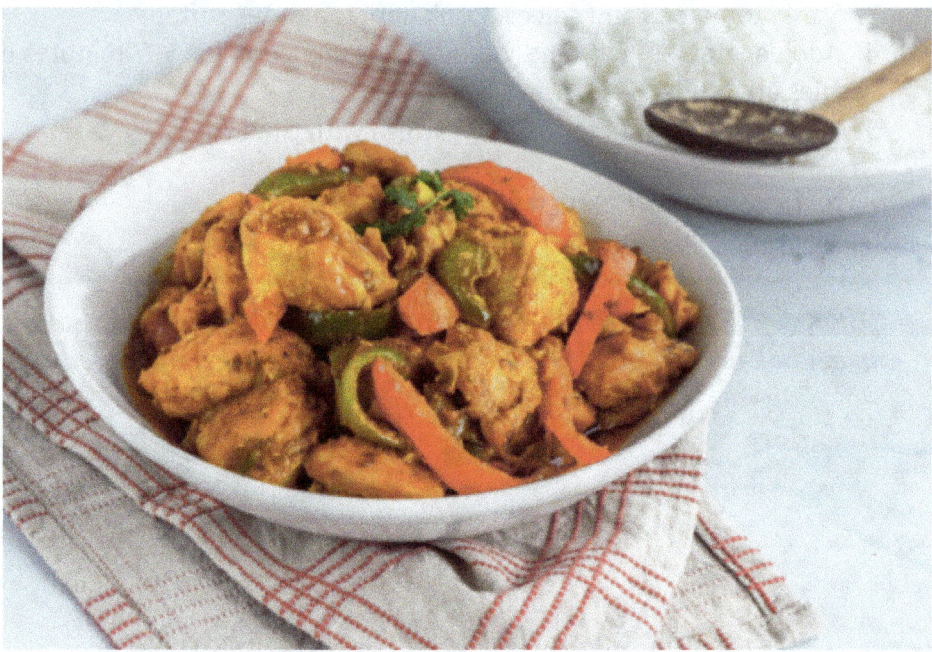

Prep Time: 5 minutes | Cook Time: 9 minutes | Makes: 2

Chicken Jalfrezi is a vibrant Indo-Chinese-style curry that features sautéed peppers, onions, and tomatoes with spiced chicken. Known for its quick stir-fry technique, this dish is perfect for busy weeknights.

INGREDIENTS:
- 250g boneless chicken, thinly sliced
- 1 tbsp oil
- 1 small onion, sliced
- ½ bell pepper, sliced
- 1 tomato, chopped
- 1 tsp ginger-garlic paste
- ½ tsp turmeric
- ½ tsp cumin powder
- ½ tsp chili powder
- ¼ tsp garam masala
- Salt, to taste
- 1 tbsp ketchup (optional)
- Chopped cilantro

INSTRUCTIONS:
1. Heat oil. Sauté onion and bell pepper for 2 minutes.

2. Add ginger-garlic paste and chicken. Stir-fry 4–5 minutes.
3. Add tomato, spices, salt, and ketchup (if using). Cook 2 more minutes.
4. Garnish with cilantro and serve with rice or naan.

NUTRITION ESTIMATES (PER SERVING):
Calories: 370 | Protein: 32g | Carbs: 9g | Fat: 23g | Fiber: 2g

QUICK & EASY TIP: *Use thin chicken strips and a high-heat pan to cook faster. Optional ketchup adds sweetness and depth quickly.*

> 58.   **Baked Tandoori Chicken Curry**

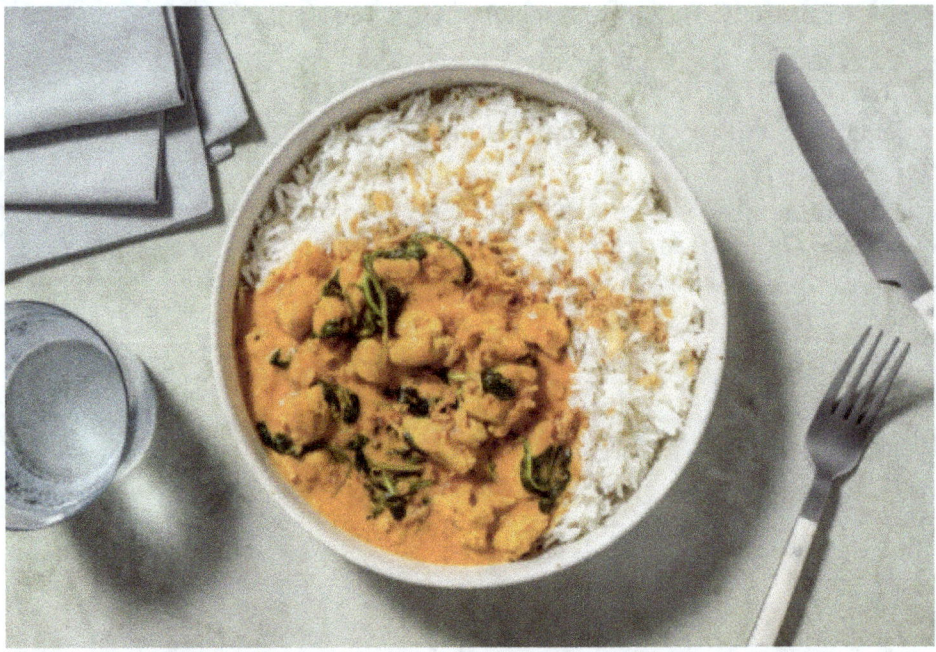

Prep Time: 5 minutes | Cook Time: 10 minutes | Makes: 2

This Baked Tandoori Chicken Curry combines the smoky flavors of traditional tandoori chicken with a creamy stovetop curry. By using pre-baked or air-fried tandoori chicken, the dish comes together in minutes.

INGREDIENTS:
- 250g pre-cooked tandoori chicken pieces
- 1 tbsp oil or ghee
- 1 small onion, finely chopped
- 1 small tomato, pureed
- 1 tsp ginger-garlic paste
- ¼ tsp turmeric
- ½ tsp cumin
- ½ tsp garam masala
- ¼ tsp chili powder
- Salt, to taste
- 3 tbsp cream or coconut milk
- Cilantro for garnish

INSTRUCTIONS:

1. Heat oil. Sauté onions until soft. Add ginger-garlic paste and cook for 30 seconds.
2. Stir in pureed tomato and spices. Cook 2–3 minutes until thickened.
3. Add cream and mix well.
4. Add pre-cooked tandoori chicken. Simmer for 3–4 minutes until heated through. Garnish with cilantro.

NUTRITION ESTIMATES (PER SERVING):
Calories: 410 | Protein: 33g | Carbs: 9g | Fat: 28g | Fiber: 2g

QUICK & EASY TIP: Bake or air-fry chicken in advance in batches and freeze. Reheat directly into curry to save time on busy nights.

59. Easy Mutton Karahi

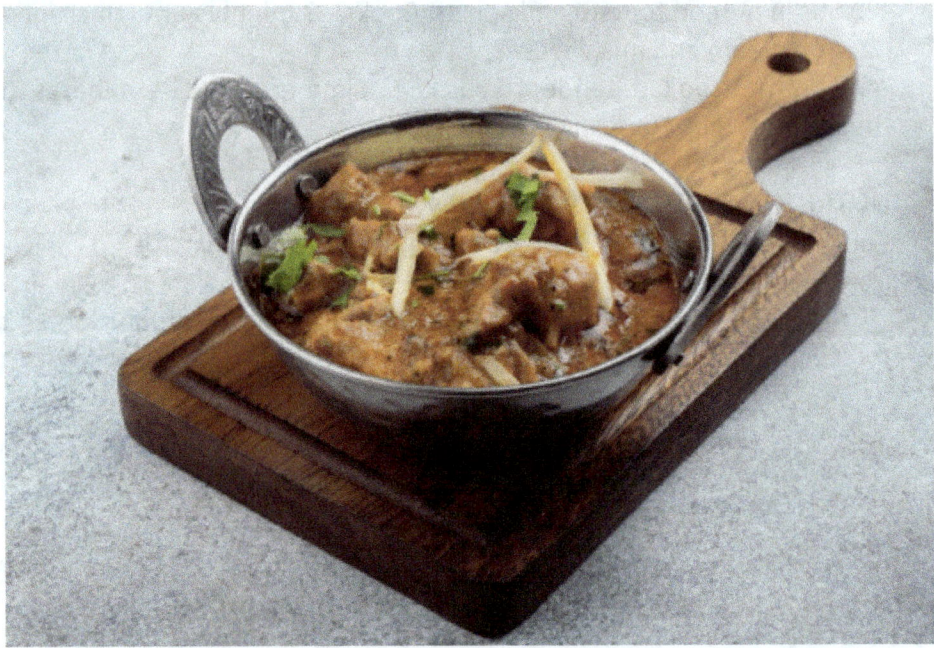

Prep Time: 5 minutes | Cook Time: 10 minutes | Makes: 2

Mutton Karahi is a robust North Indian and Pakistani curry made with mutton, tomatoes, and ginger. Traditionally slow-cooked, this express version uses thinly sliced or pre-cooked mutton to deliver rich flavor in minutes.

INGREDIENTS:
- 250g thinly sliced or pre-cooked mutton
- 1 tbsp oil or ghee
- 1 small onion, finely sliced
- 2 tomatoes, chopped
- 1 tsp ginger-garlic paste
- ½ tsp cumin
- ½ tsp chili powder
- ½ tsp coriander powder
- Salt, to taste
- ¼ tsp garam masala
- Fresh ginger and green chili, for garnish

INSTRUCTIONS:
1. Heat oil in a karahi or pan. Sauté onions until lightly browned.

2. Add ginger-garlic paste, cook 30 seconds. Add tomatoes and spices. Cook 2–3 minutes until soft.
3. Add mutton. Sauté and stir until coated and heated through (5 minutes).
4. Garnish with sliced ginger and green chili.

NUTRITION ESTIMATES (PER SERVING):
Calories: 420 | Protein: 31g | Carbs: 9g | Fat: 29g | Fiber: 2g

QUICK & EASY TIP: Use thin mutton slices or pressure-cooked leftovers to reduce cook time dramatically. Keep the base simple for speed.

60. Indian Fish Curry

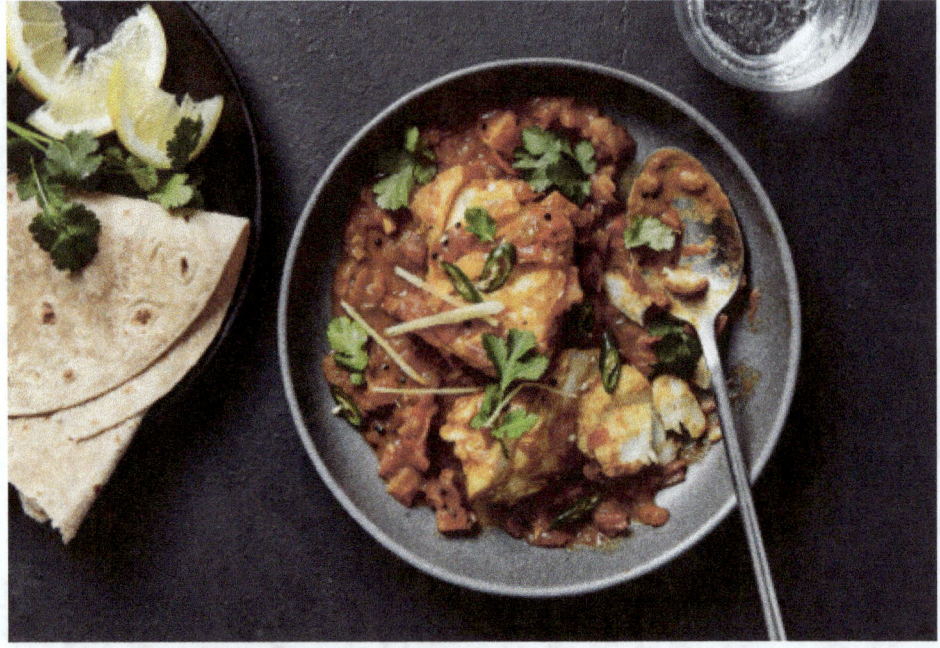

Prep Time: 4 minutes | Cook Time: 10 minutes | Makes: 2

Fish Masala Curry is a coastal classic, loved for its tangy-spicy tomato base and fast cooking time. This version works beautifully with boneless fillets like tilapia or cod, making it ideal for quick dinners.

INGREDIENTS:
- 250g firm white fish fillets (cubed)
- 1 tbsp oil
- 1 small onion, chopped
- 1 tomato, pureed
- 1 tsp ginger-garlic paste
- ½ tsp turmeric
- ½ tsp red chili powder
- ½ tsp coriander powder
- Salt, to taste
- ¼ tsp mustard seeds (optional)
- ½ tsp garam masala
- Chopped cilantro for garnish

INSTRUCTIONS:
1. Heat oil. Add mustard seeds (if using) and let them splutter.

2. Sauté onion for 2–3 minutes. Add ginger-garlic paste and cook briefly.
3. Add tomato puree and spices. Cook for 2–3 minutes until thickened.
4. Gently add fish cubes and simmer for 4–5 minutes until cooked through.
5. Finish with garam masala and garnish with cilantro.

NUTRITION ESTIMATES (PER SERVING):
Calories: 310 | Protein: 32g | Carbs: 7g | Fat: 18g | Fiber: 1g

QUICK & EASY TIP: *Use boneless fish fillets to reduce cooking time. Avoid stirring too much after adding fish to keep pieces intact.*

THAI DINNERS

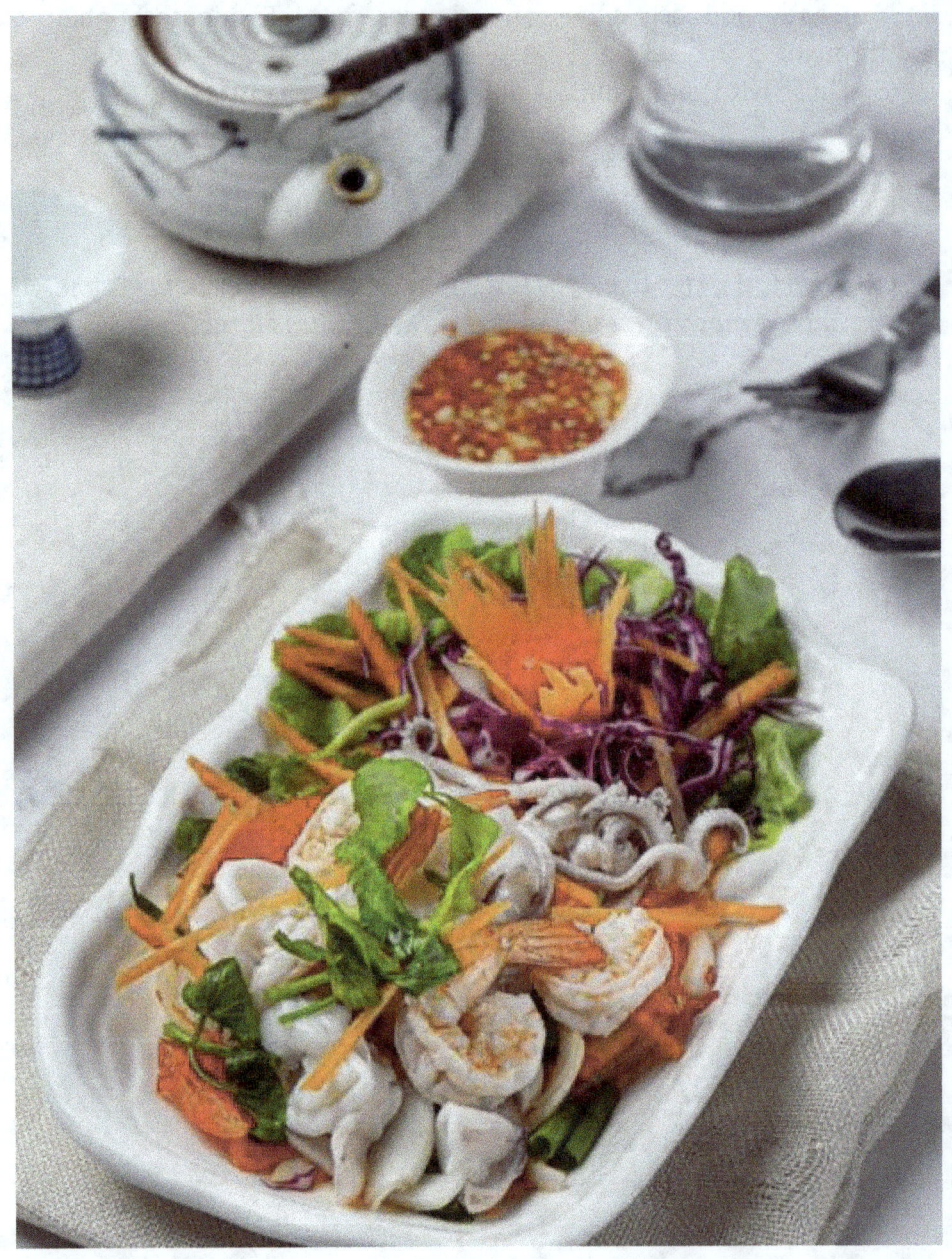

61. Pad Kra Pao (Thai Basil Chicken)

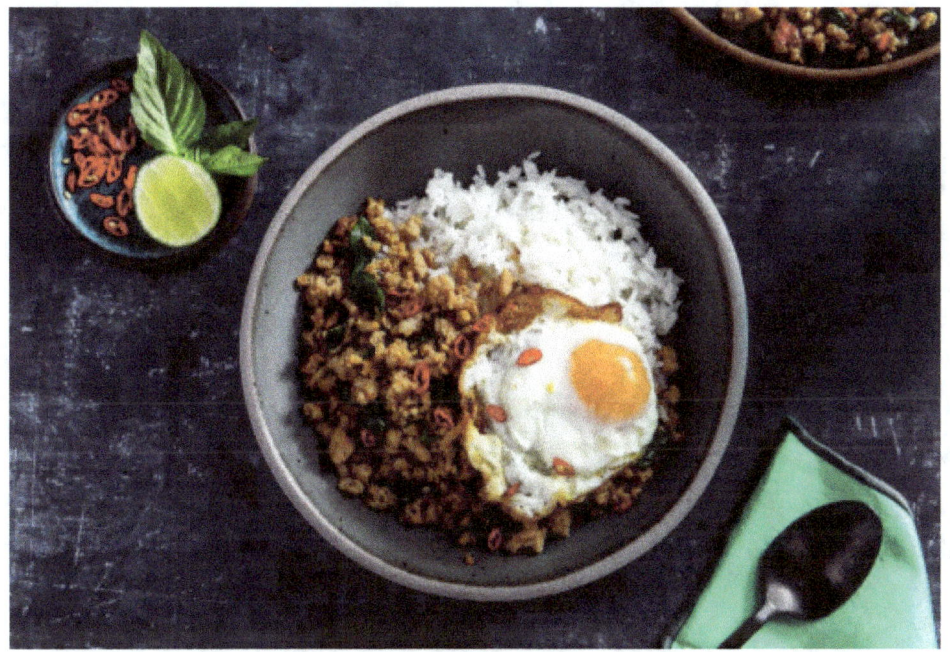

Prep Time: 5 minutes | Cook Time: 10 minutes | Makes: 2

This beloved Thai street food features ground chicken stir-fried with garlic, chili, and Thai basil. It's spicy, aromatic, and perfect with jasmine rice.

INGREDIENTS:
- 250g ground chicken
- 1 tbsp vegetable oil
- 3 garlic cloves, minced
- 1 red chili, finely sliced (adjust to heat preference)
- 1 tbsp oyster sauce
- 1 tbsp soy sauce
- 1 tsp fish sauce
- 1/2 tsp sugar
- 1/2 cup fresh Thai basil leaves
- Cooked jasmine rice, to serve
- Fried egg (optional), to top

INSTRUCTIONS:
1. Heat oil in a wok or pan. Add garlic and chili. Sauté for 30 seconds.
2. Add ground chicken. Stir-fry until browned, 5–6 minutes.
3. Add oyster sauce, soy sauce, fish sauce, and sugar. Stir well.

4. Toss in basil leaves. Stir until wilted.
5. Serve over rice, topped with a fried egg if desired.

NUTRITION ESTIMATES (PER SERVING):
Calories: 390 | Protein: 30g | Carbs: 20g | Fat: 22g

<u>*QUICK & EASY TIP:*</u> *Use pre-ground chicken and ready rice packs to speed up dinner even more.*

62. Thai Shrimp Red Curry

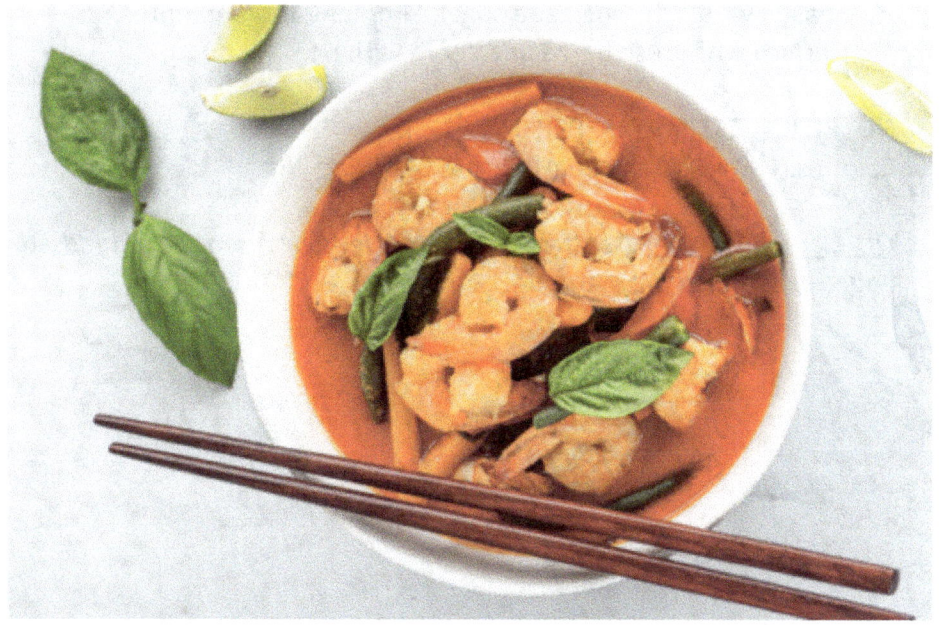

Prep Time: 5 minutes | Cook Time: 10 minutes | Makes: 2

Thai red curry is a cornerstone of Thai cuisine, known for its fiery heat, aromatic herbs, and creamy coconut base. Originating from central Thailand, this dish balances spice, sweetness, and saltiness — a signature of Thai flavor harmony. Red curry paste (prik gaeng ped) is traditionally made with red chilies, lemongrass, garlic, and galangal, and was once pounded by hand with a mortar and pestle. Today, it's a weeknight hero — bold, quick, and deeply satisfying.

INGREDIENTS:
- 200g shrimp, peeled and deveined
- 1 tbsp red curry paste
- 1/2 can (200ml) coconut milk
- 1 tbsp vegetable oil
- 1/2 red bell pepper, sliced
- 1/2 zucchini, sliced
- 1 tsp fish sauce
- 1/2 tsp sugar
- Fresh basil or cilantro, to garnish
- Cooked jasmine rice, to serve

INSTRUCTIONS:
1. Heat oil in a skillet. Add curry paste and fry for 30 seconds.

2. Pour in coconut milk. Stir until smooth and simmer for 2 minutes.
3. Add shrimp, bell pepper, and zucchini. Cook for 5–6 minutes.
4. Season with fish sauce and sugar. Simmer 1 more minute.
5. Garnish with fresh herbs and serve with rice.

NUTRITION ESTIMATES (PER SERVING):
Calories: 400 | Protein: 26g | Carbs: 14g | Fat: 28g

QUICK & EASY TIP: *Use frozen, pre-peeled shrimp and bagged stir-fry vegetables to cut prep time.*

63. Thai Glass Noodle Stir-Fry (Pad Woon Sen)

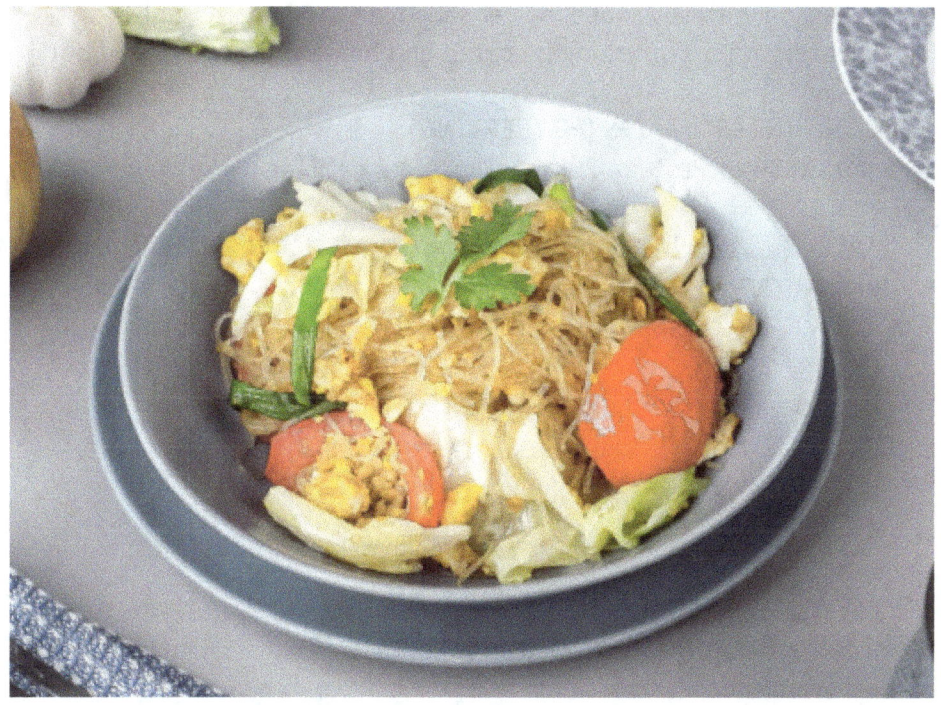

Prep Time: 5 minutes | Cook Time: 10 minutes | Makes: 2

Pad Woon Sen is a beloved Thai noodle dish made with glass noodles, veggies, and protein, stir-fried in a sweet-savory sauce. Light yet satisfying.

INGREDIENTS:
- 100g glass noodles (soaked in warm water for 5 minutes)
- 1 tbsp vegetable oil
- 1 egg, beaten
- 1 small carrot, julienned
- 1/2 onion, sliced
- 1/2 cup shredded cabbage
- 1/2 cup cooked chicken or shrimp
- 1 tbsp soy sauce
- 1 tbsp oyster sauce
- 1/2 tsp sugar
- Black pepper, to taste

INSTRUCTIONS:
1. Heat oil in a wok. Add egg and scramble until set.

2. Add onion, carrot, and cabbage. Stir-fry for 2–3 minutes.
3. Add protein of choice and drained noodles.
4. Season with soy sauce, oyster sauce, and sugar. Toss well.
5. Stir-fry until everything is coated and heated through. Serve hot.

NUTRITION ESTIMATES (PER SERVING):
Calories: 360 | Protein: 20g | Carbs: 40g | Fat: 14g

QUICK & EASY TIP: *Use pre-cooked protein and pre-cut veggies for quicker prep.*

| 64. | Thai Chicken Lettuce Wraps |

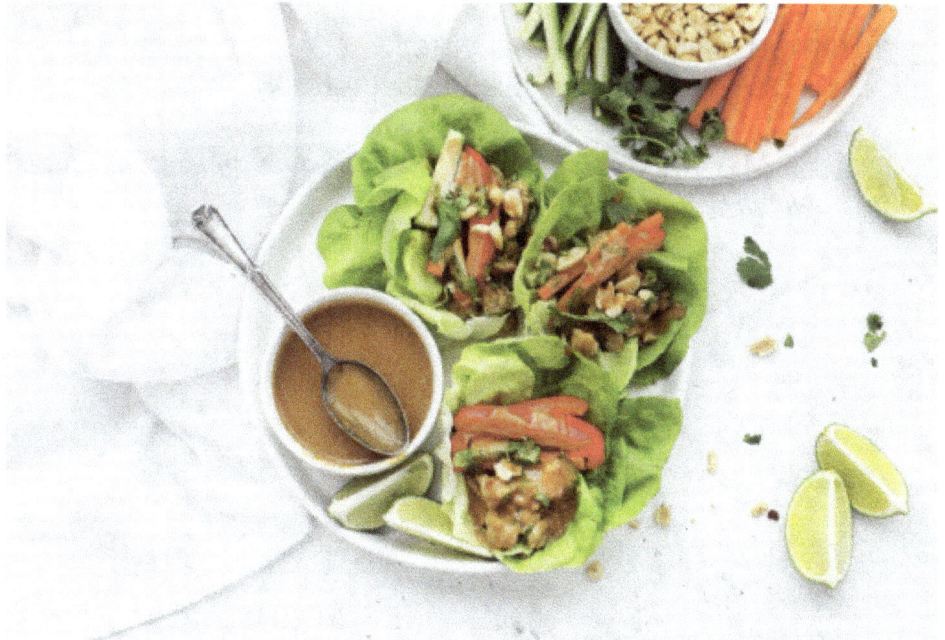

Prep Time: 5 minutes | Cook Time: 10 minutes | Makes: 2

A lighter, low-carb Thai dinner with ground chicken seasoned in savory Thai spices, served in crisp lettuce cups—fresh, fast, and full of flavor.

INGREDIENTS:
- 250g ground chicken
- 1 tbsp vegetable oil
- 2 garlic cloves, minced
- 1/2 red chili, minced (optional)
- 1 tbsp soy sauce
- 1 tbsp oyster sauce
- 1 tsp fish sauce
- 1/2 tsp sugar
- Juice of 1/2 lime
- Butter lettuce leaves, to serve
- Chopped peanuts and cilantro, for garnish

INSTRUCTIONS:
1. Heat oil in a skillet. Add garlic and chili. Sauté for 30 seconds.
2. Add chicken. Cook until browned, about 6–7 minutes.
3. Stir in soy sauce, oyster sauce, fish sauce, sugar, and lime juice.

4. Spoon into lettuce cups. Garnish with peanuts and cilantro. Serve immediately.

NUTRITION ESTIMATES (PER SERVING):
Calories: 330 | Protein: 28g | Carbs: 10g | Fat: 20g

QUICK & EASY TIP: Use pre-washed lettuce leaves and ground chicken to cut down on time.

65. Tom Yum Soup (Thai Hot and Sour Soup)

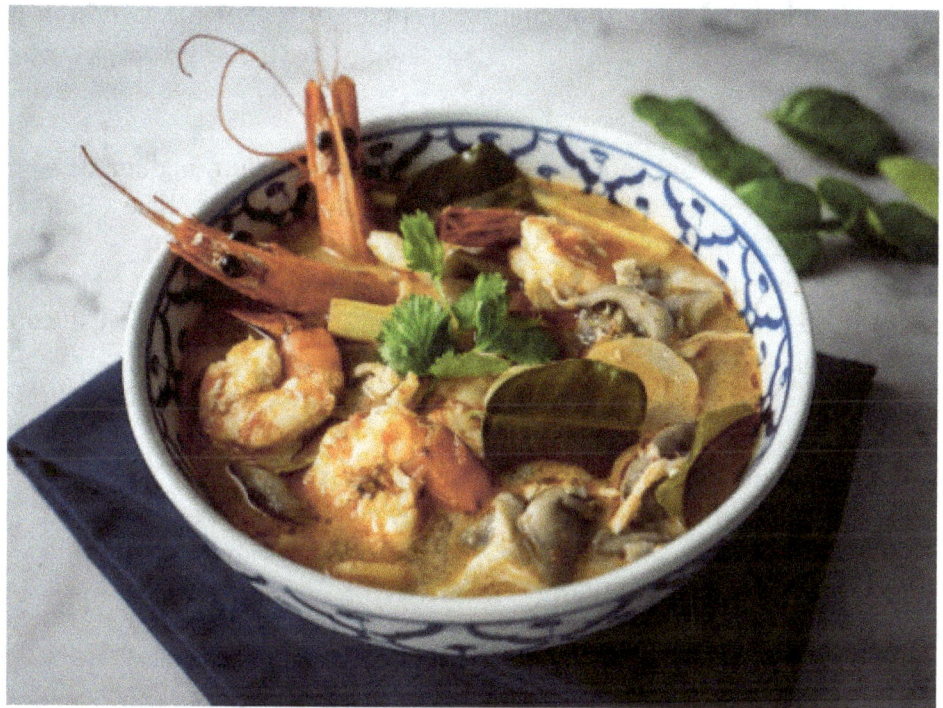

Prep Time: 5 minutes | Cook Time: 10 minutes | Serves: 2

Tom Yum, Thailand's iconic hot and sour soup, has been a culinary staple since at least the 19th century. Believed to originate from Central Thailand, this dish is prized for its harmony of flavors—spicy chilies, sour lime, fragrant herbs, and umami from fish sauce or shrimp. Traditionally made with river prawns (Tom Yum Goong), it reflects the Thai philosophy of balance and simplicity, often served in homes and street stalls alike.

INGREDIENTS:
- 2 cups water or chicken broth
- 6 medium shrimp, peeled and deveined
- 2 stalks lemongrass, cut into 2-inch pieces and smashed
- 3 kaffir lime leaves, torn into pieces
- 3–4 thin slices galangal (or ginger if unavailable)
- 1 small shallot, sliced
- 4–5 white or brown mushrooms, sliced
- 1 small tomato, cut into wedges
- 2 Thai bird's eye chilies (or to taste), smashed
- 2 tbsp fish sauce
- 1½ tbsp lime juice (or more to taste)

- ½ tsp sugar
- Fresh cilantro, for garnish
- (Optional: 1 tbsp Thai chili paste (nam prik pao) for Tom Yum Nam Khon style)

INSTRUCTIONS:
1. Bring water or broth to a boil in a pot over medium-high heat.
2. Add lemongrass, lime leaves, galangal, shallots, and chilies. Boil for 2–3 minutes to infuse.
3. Add mushrooms and tomato. Simmer for 2 minutes.
4. Add shrimp and cook for 2–3 minutes until pink and just cooked through.
5. Stir in fish sauce, lime juice, and sugar. Taste and adjust saltiness or sourness if needed.
6. (Optional) Stir in chili paste for a richer broth.
7. Remove from heat, garnish with fresh cilantro, and serve hot.

NUTRITION INFORMATION (PER SERVING):
Calories: 160 | Protein: 16g | Carbs: 6g | Fat: 8g | Fiber: 1g

<u>QUICK & EASY TIP:</u> Pre-peeled frozen shrimp and lemongrass paste help reduce prep time. Leftover broth can double as a quick noodle base for another meal.

MIDDLE EASTERN DINNERS

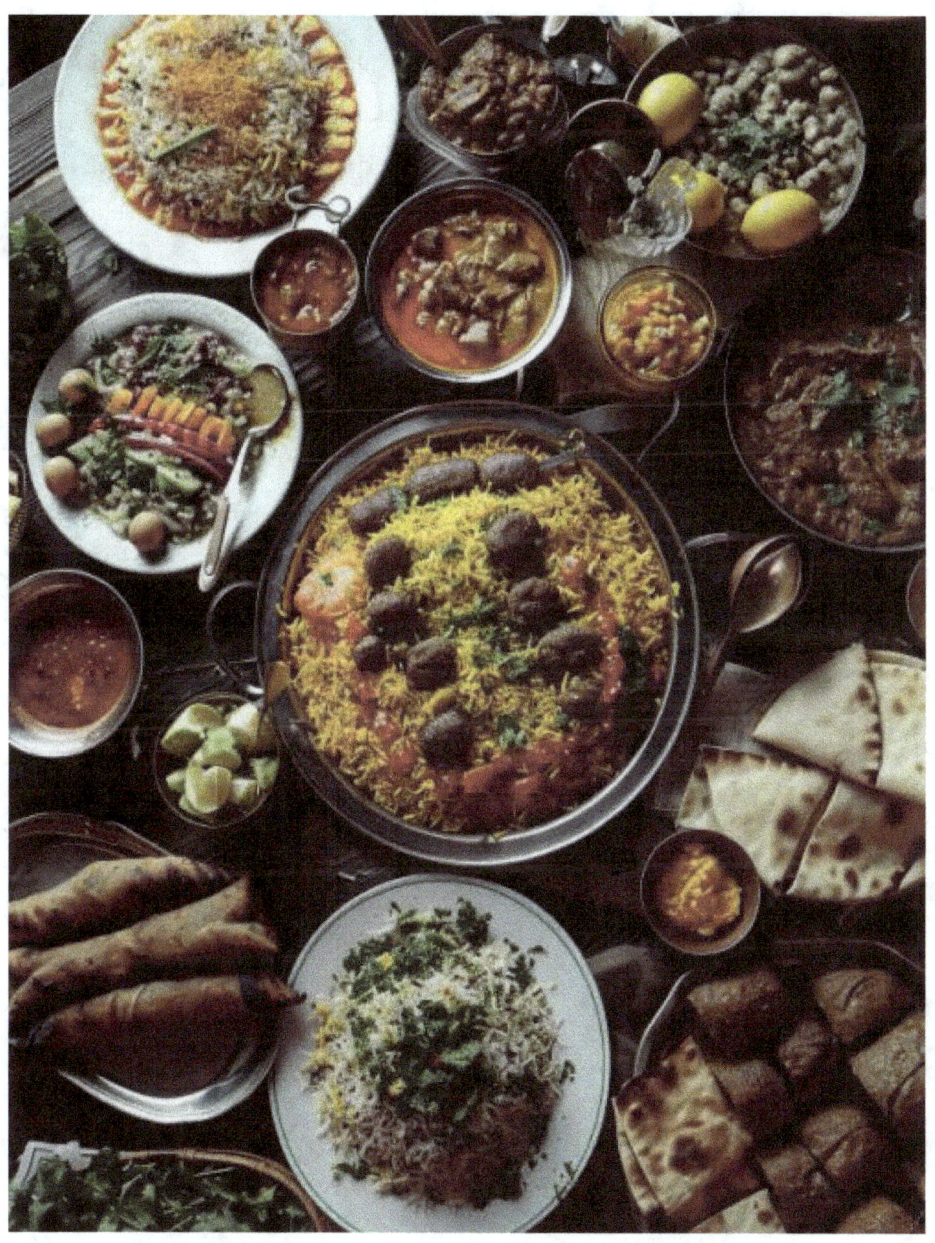

66. Chicken Shawarma Wrap Bowls

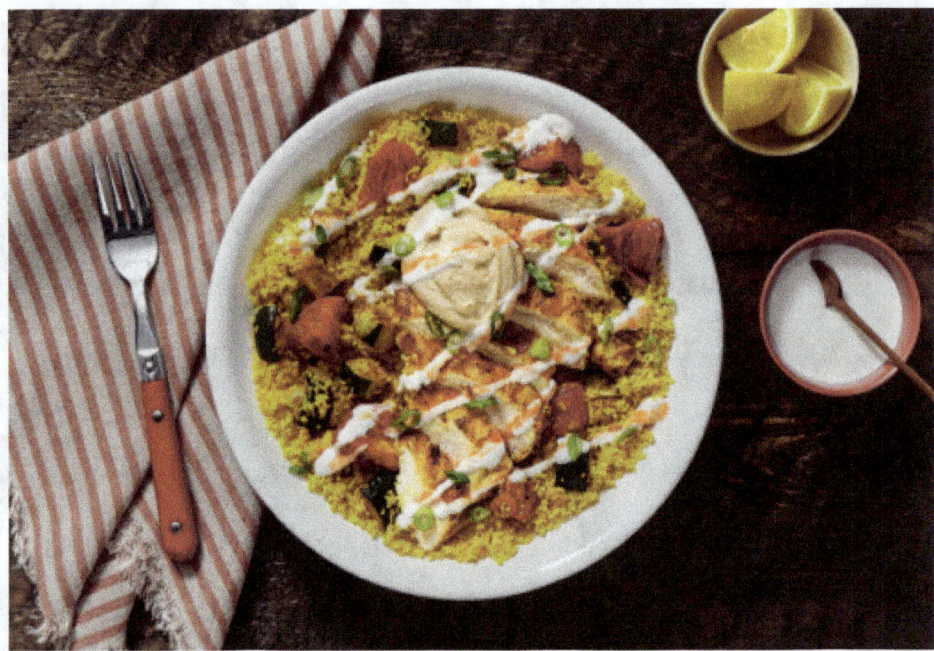

Prep Time: 5 minutes | Cook Time: 10 minutes | Makes: 2

Shawarma is a cornerstone of Middle Eastern street food — typically cooked on vertical rotisseries. This fast skillet version delivers all the flavor in a fraction of the time, using sliced chicken, warm spices, and a simple yogurt drizzle. Served deconstructed in a bowl, it's a modern, dinner-friendly twist.

INGREDIENTS:
- 200g boneless chicken breast or thigh, thinly sliced
- 1 tbsp olive oil
- ½ tsp ground cumin
- ½ tsp paprika
- ½ tsp garlic powder
- ¼ tsp cinnamon
- Salt and pepper, to taste
- 1 cup cooked rice or couscous
- ½ cup chopped cucumber
- ½ cup cherry tomatoes, halved
- 2 tbsp plain yogurt
- ½ tsp lemon juice
- Optional: chopped parsley or mint

INSTRUCTIONS:
1. In a bowl, toss chicken with olive oil, cumin, paprika, garlic powder, cinnamon, salt, and pepper.
2. Heat a skillet over medium-high heat. Sear chicken for 4–5 minutes per side until fully cooked and browned.
3. While chicken cooks, prep the bowl: divide rice, cucumber, and tomatoes between two bowls.
4. Stir lemon juice into yogurt for a quick drizzle sauce.
5. Top bowls with hot chicken and spoon over yogurt sauce. Garnish with herbs.

NUTRITION ESTIMATES (PER SERVING):
Calories: 460 | Protein: 35g | Carbs: 34g | Fat: 21g | Fiber: 3g

QUICK & EASY TIP: Use pre-cooked or leftover rice to save time.

67. Spiced Lamb and Eggplant Skillet

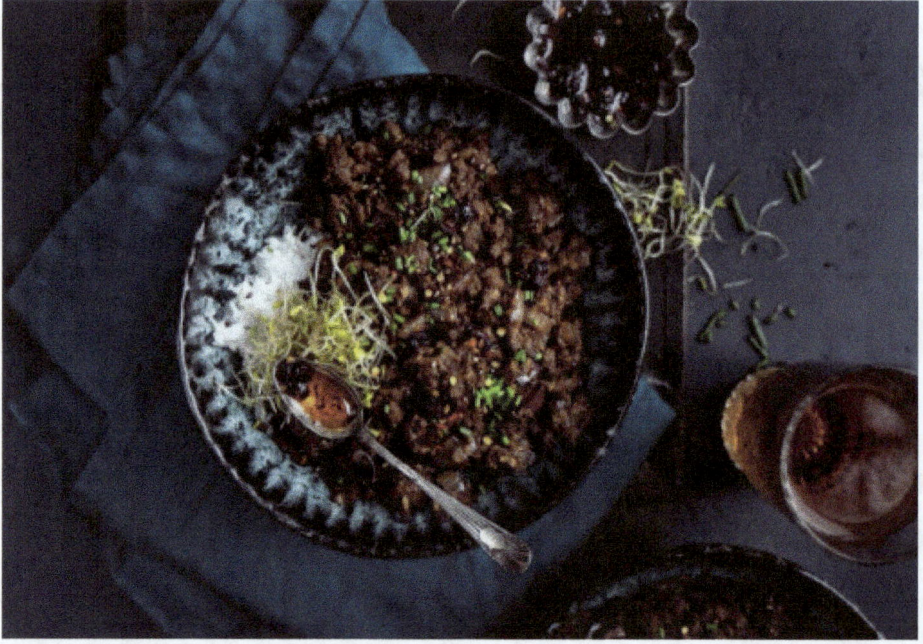

Prep Time: 5 minutes | Cook Time: 10 minutes | Makes: 2

This hearty lamb and eggplant dish draws from Levantine and Persian cooking, where warming spices and vegetables are often cooked together in one pan. It's rich, savory, and perfect for dinner when you want depth of flavor fast — no oven or long simmering needed.

INGREDIENTS:
- 200g ground lamb
- 1 tbsp olive oil
- 1 small eggplant, diced small
- 1 garlic clove, minced
- ½ tsp ground coriander
- ½ tsp cumin
- ¼ tsp cinnamon
- Salt and pepper, to taste
- 1 tbsp tomato paste
- ¼ cup water
- Optional: chopped parsley, warm pita, or couscous for serving

INSTRUCTIONS:

1. Heat oil in a skillet over medium heat. Add lamb and cook for 3–4 minutes, breaking it up as it browns.
2. Add eggplant and garlic. Stir in coriander, cumin, cinnamon, salt, and pepper. Cook 4–5 minutes, until eggplant is soft.
3. Stir in tomato paste and water. Simmer 1–2 minutes to create a light sauce.
4. Serve hot with parsley and optional pita or couscous.

NUTRITION ESTIMATES (PER SERVING):
Calories: 490 | Protein: 25g | Carbs: 14g | Fat: 36g | Fiber: 4g

QUICK & EASY TIP: Dice eggplant small to speed up cooking and avoid pre-roasting.

68. Za'atar Chicken with Hummus and Pita

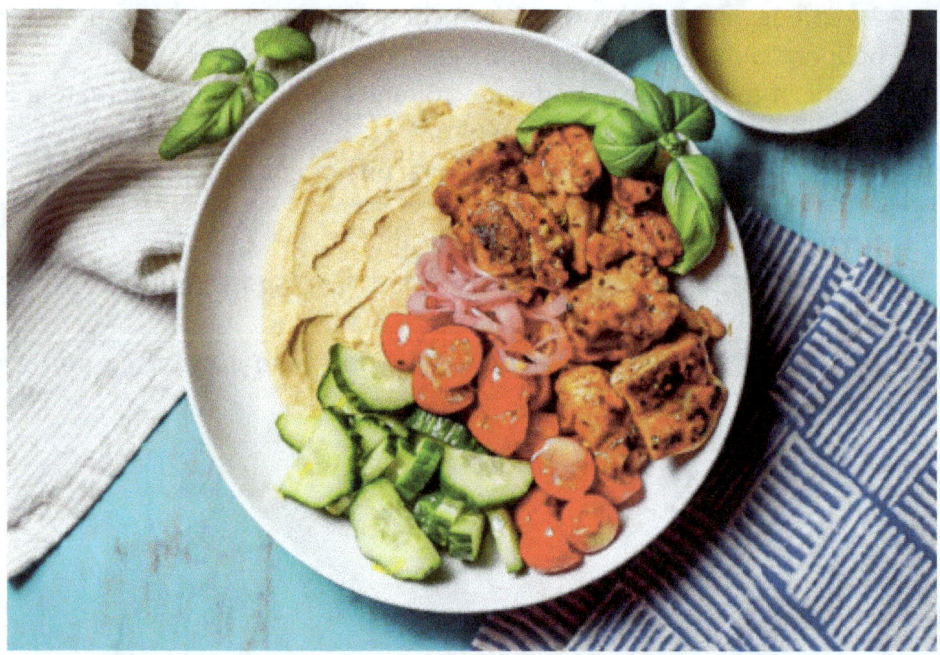

Prep Time: 5 minutes | Cook Time: 10 minutes | Makes: 2

Za'atar — a fragrant herb and spice blend — is a staple across Levantine cuisine. This dish pairs za'atar-crusted chicken with creamy hummus and warm pita for a satisfying, protein-rich dinner. Popular in Lebanese and Palestinian homes, it's often eaten with hands, wrapped, or dipped.

INGREDIENTS:
- 2 boneless chicken breasts, pounded thin
- 1 tbsp olive oil
- 1 tbsp za'atar spice blend
- Salt, to taste
- ½ cup hummus
- 2 pita breads, warmed
- ½ cup cherry tomatoes, halved
- ¼ cup sliced cucumbers
- Lemon wedges, to serve

INSTRUCTIONS:
1. Rub chicken with olive oil, za'atar, and salt.
2. Heat a skillet over medium-high heat. Sear chicken 4–5 minutes per side until golden and cooked through.
3. Plate with a dollop of hummus, pita on the side, and fresh veggies.

4. Serve with lemon wedges and optional extra za'atar drizzle.

NUTRITION ESTIMATES (PER SERVING):
Calories: 520 | Protein: 40g | Carbs: 28g | Fat: 28g | Fiber: 5g

QUICK & EASY TIP: Use store-bought hummus and pre-sliced veggies for a no-prep finish.

| 69. | Chickpea and Spinach Stew |

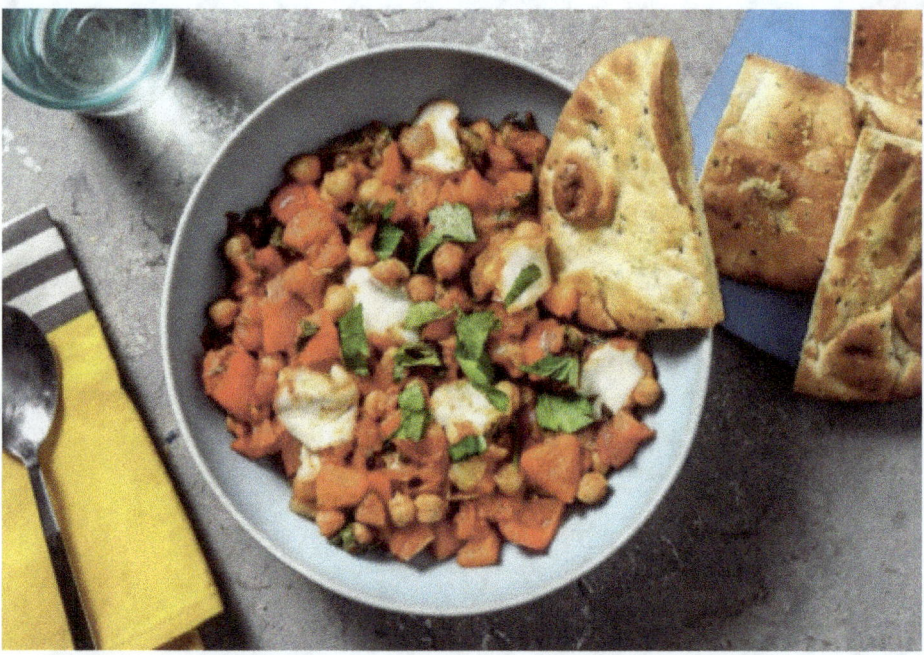

Prep Time: 5 minutes | Cook Time: 10 minutes | Makes: 2

Inspired by Syrian and Egyptian kitchens, this fast chickpea and spinach stew is nourishing, filling, and naturally vegan. Commonly enjoyed with flatbread or rice, it's seasoned with garlic, cumin, and lemon — simple pantry ingredients transformed into a warm, comforting meal.

INGREDIENTS:
- 1 tbsp olive oil
- 1 garlic clove, minced
- 1 tsp ground cumin
- 1 cup canned chickpeas, drained
- 2 cups spinach leaves (or 1 cup frozen)
- ¼ tsp chili flakes (optional)
- Salt and pepper, to taste
- ½ cup vegetable broth or water
- Juice of ½ lemon
- Flatbread or rice, to serve

INSTRUCTIONS:

1. Heat olive oil in a pan over medium heat. Add garlic and cumin, sauté for 30 seconds.
2. Add chickpeas and chili flakes. Cook 2 minutes.
3. Add spinach and broth. Simmer for 5–6 minutes until spinach wilts and flavors combine.
4. Finish with lemon juice, season to taste, and serve hot with bread or rice.

NUTRITION ESTIMATES (PER SERVING):
Calories: 350 | Protein: 13g | Carbs: 34g | Fat: 18g | Fiber: 9g

QUICK & EASY TIP: Use canned chickpeas and pre-washed spinach to skip all prep.

70. Kofta Rice Bowl with Tahini

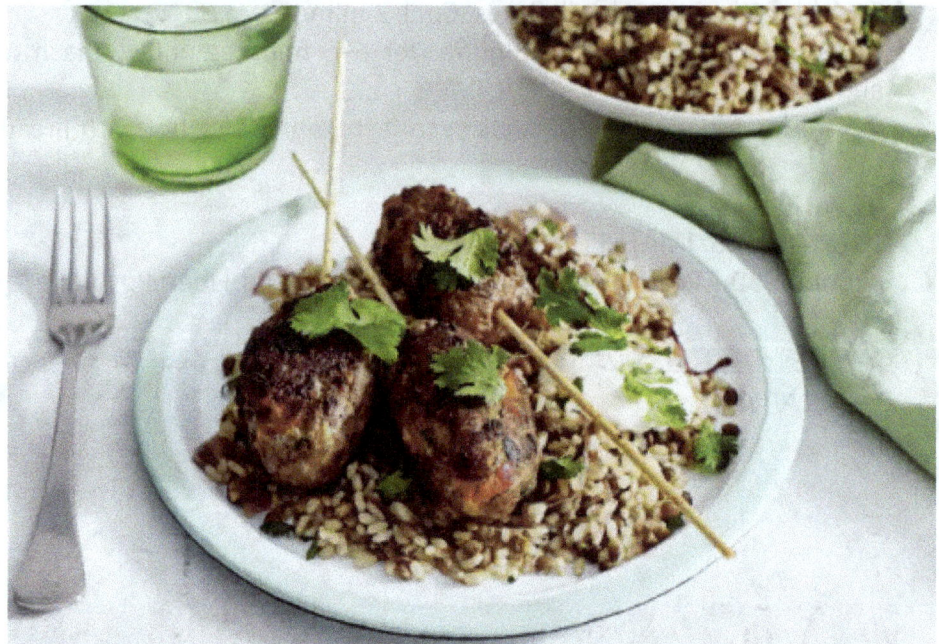

Prep Time: 5 minutes | Cook Time: 10 minutes | Makes: 2

Kofta — spiced ground meat shaped into logs or patties — is a beloved staple from Egypt to Iran. This simplified skillet version turns them into fast, juicy patties served over rice with a lemony tahini sauce. A complete dinner that feels indulgent but comes together quickly.

INGREDIENTS:
- 200g ground beef or lamb
- 1 tbsp finely chopped onion
- 1 garlic clove, minced
- ½ tsp ground cumin
- ½ tsp ground coriander
- Salt and pepper, to taste
- 1 tsp oil
- 1 cup cooked rice
- 2 tbsp tahini
- 1 tbsp lemon juice
- 2 tbsp water
- Chopped parsley, for garnish

INSTRUCTIONS:

1. In a bowl, mix ground meat, onion, garlic, cumin, coriander, salt, and pepper. Shape into 4–6 small patties.
2. Heat oil in a skillet over medium heat. Cook koftas 3–4 minutes per side until browned and cooked through.
3. In a small bowl, whisk tahini, lemon juice, and water until smooth.
4. Plate rice, top with koftas, drizzle with tahini sauce, and garnish with parsley.

NUTRITION ESTIMATES (PER SERVING):
Calories: 510 | Protein: 28g | Carbs: 32g | Fat: 30g | Fiber: 3g

QUICK & EASY TIP: *Use pre-cooked rice and mix koftas ahead to reduce active cooking time.*

71.   Ful Medames with Fried Egg and Pita

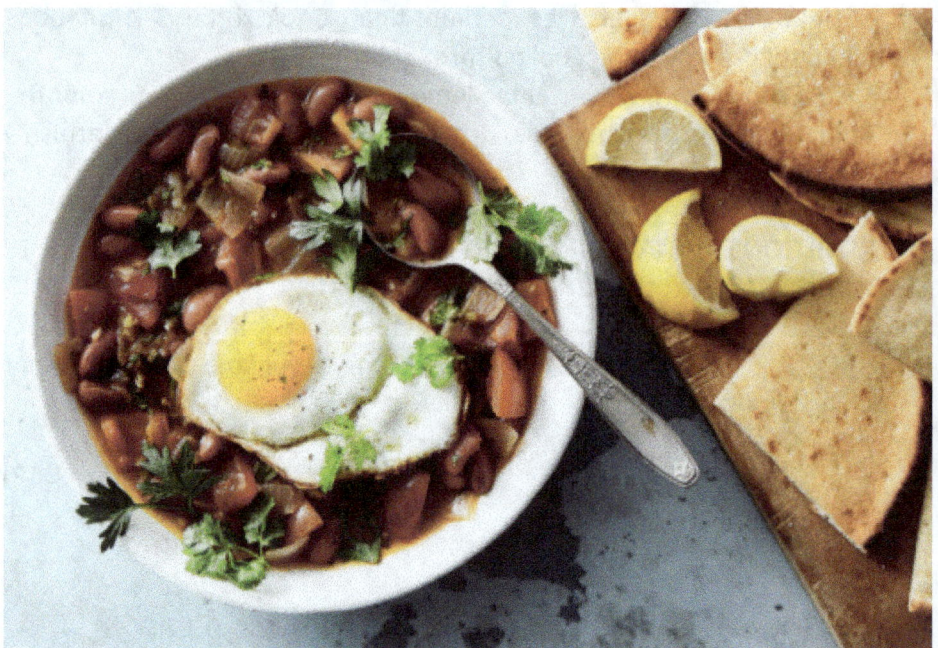

Prep Time: 3 minutes | Cook Time: 10 minutes | Makes: 2

Ful Medames, made with fava beans, is Egypt's national dish — a hearty, humble staple eaten for breakfast, lunch, or dinner. This speedy version combines canned beans with olive oil, cumin, and lemon, topped with a fried egg for a protein boost and dinner-worthy richness.

INGREDIENTS:
- 1 tbsp olive oil
- 1 garlic clove, minced
- 1 can (400g) fava beans, drained
- ½ tsp cumin
- Salt and pepper, to taste
- Juice of ½ lemon
- 2 eggs
- 2 pita breads, warmed
- Optional: parsley, chili flakes, chopped tomato

INSTRUCTIONS:
1. In a saucepan, heat olive oil and sauté garlic for 30 seconds. Add beans, cumin, salt, and pepper. Simmer 5–6 minutes, mashing slightly.
2. Meanwhile, fry eggs in a nonstick pan to your preference.

3. Stir lemon juice into beans. Divide between plates and top each with a fried egg.
4. Serve with warm pita and optional toppings.

NUTRITION ESTIMATES (PER SERVING):
Calories: 460 | Protein: 21g | Carbs: 38g | Fat: 24g | Fiber: 9g

<u>QUICK & EASY TIP</u>: Canned fava beans are fully cooked — just reheat and season.

EUROPEAN DINNERS

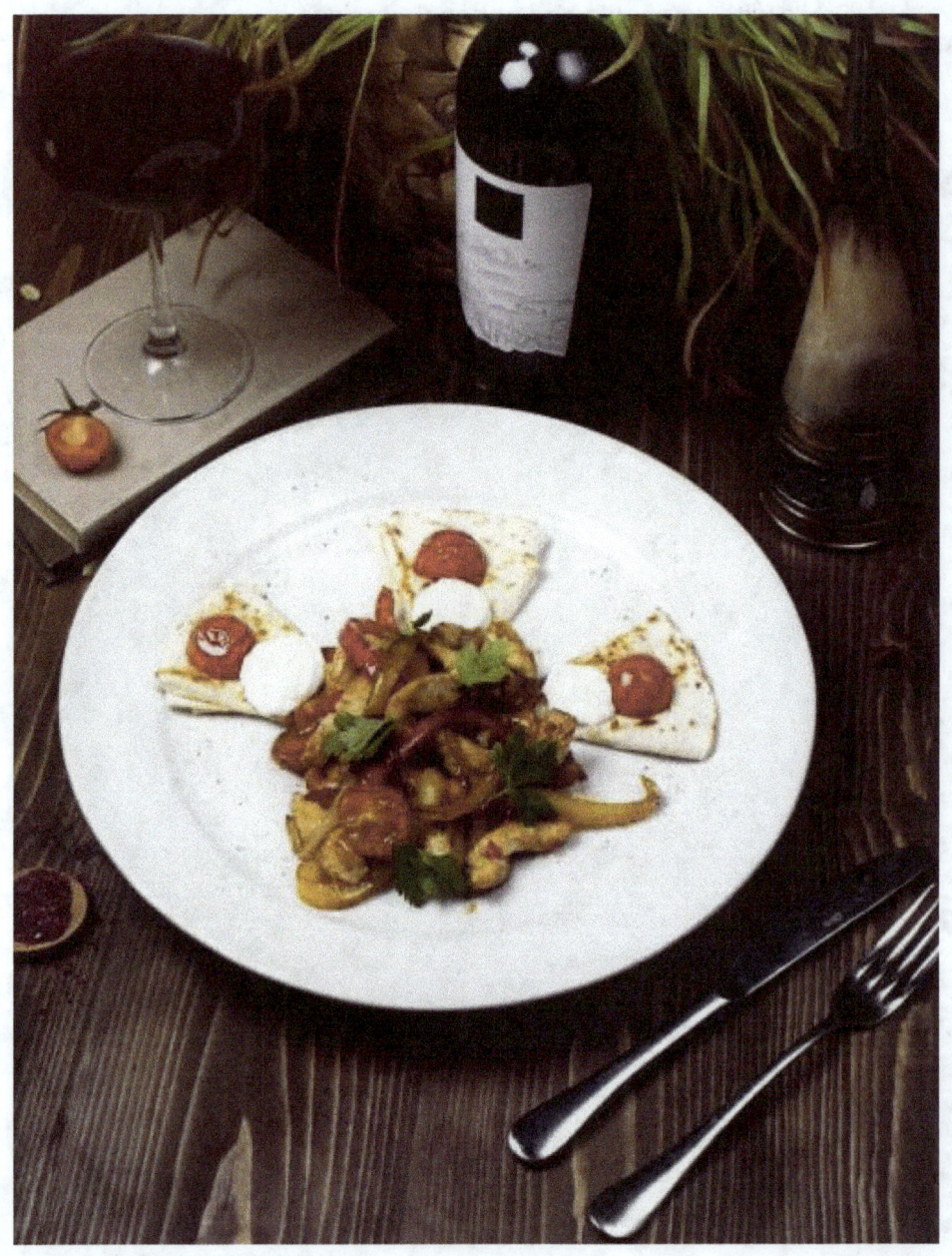

72. Scandinavian Salmon with Dill Yogurt Sauce

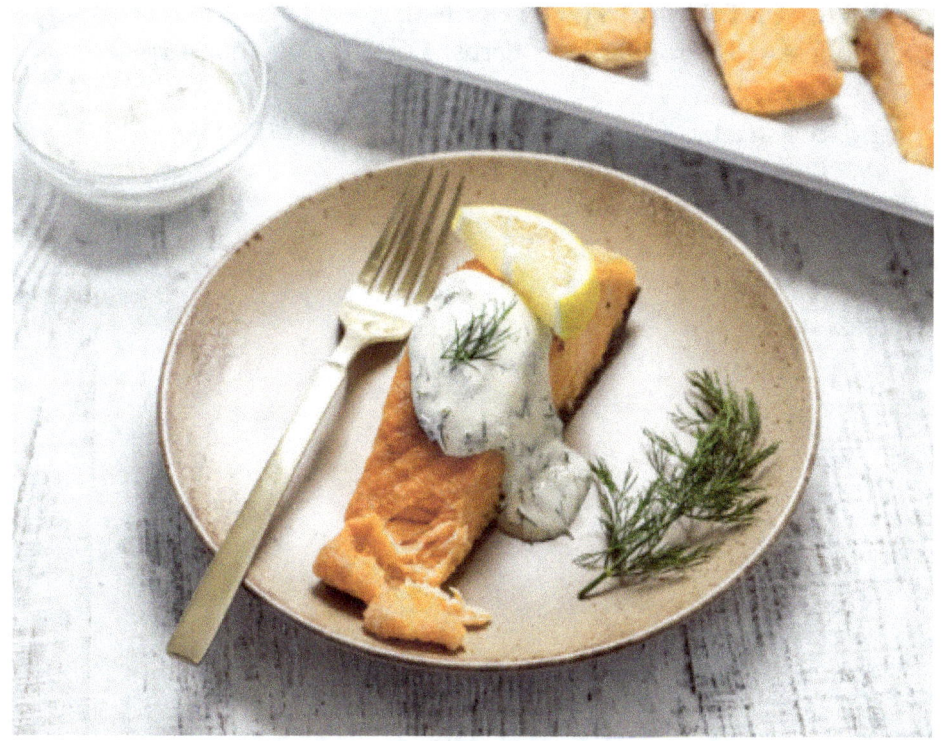

Prep Time: 5 minutes | Cook Time: 10 minutes | Makes: 2

This Nordic-inspired dish pairs pan-seared salmon with a cooling yogurt-dill sauce — a classic combination in Scandinavian home cooking. It's fresh, high-protein, and ideal for a quick, wholesome dinner. Traditionally served with potatoes, this version swaps in leafy greens for speed.

INGREDIENTS:
- 2 salmon fillets (about 150g each)
- 1 tbsp olive oil
- Salt and black pepper, to taste
- ¼ cup plain Greek yogurt
- 1 tbsp fresh or dried dill
- 1 tsp lemon juice
- 2 cups arugula or baby spinach, to serve

INSTRUCTIONS:
1. Season salmon with salt and pepper.
2. Heat oil in a nonstick skillet over medium-high heat. Cook salmon 4–5 minutes per side until golden and flaky.
3. Meanwhile, mix yogurt, dill, and lemon juice in a bowl.

4. Plate salmon over greens and spoon yogurt sauce on top.

NUTRITION ESTIMATES (PER SERVING):
Calories: 410 | Protein: 35g | Carbs: 4g | Fat: 27g | Fiber: 1g

<u>*QUICK & EASY TIP:*</u> *Salmon cooks fastest when brought to room temp — take it out while prepping sauce.*

73. German Pork Schnitzel with Lemon and Greens

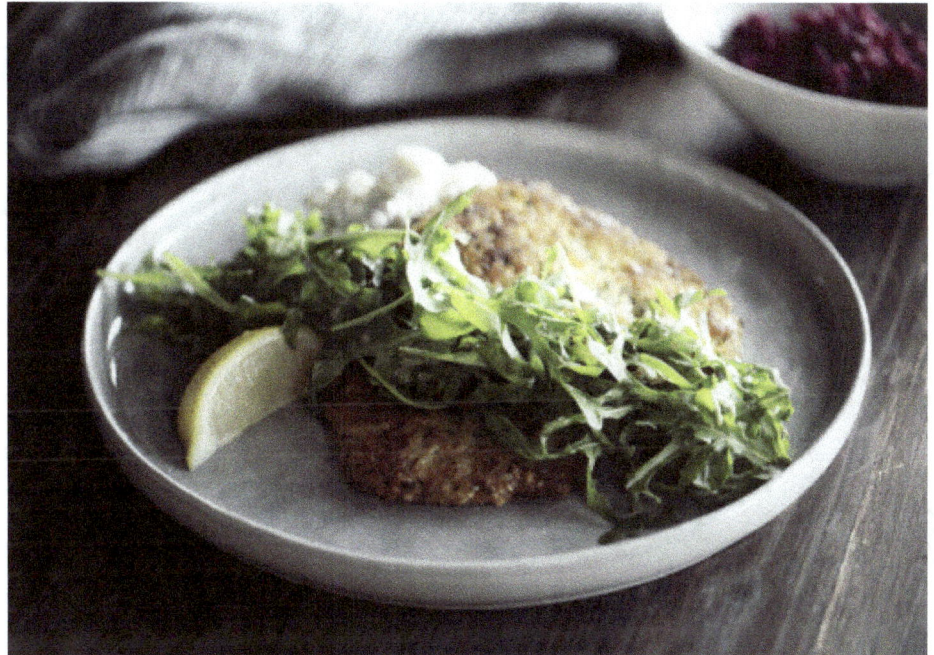

Prep Time: 5 minutes | Cook Time: 10 minutes | Makes: 2

Few dishes are as iconic in Central Europe as schnitzel. While its origins trace back to Austria's Wiener Schnitzel made with veal, the German version typically uses pork — more accessible and just as delicious. Introduced in the 19th century, schnitzel quickly became a comfort food favorite in German households, restaurants, and beer halls alike. It's often enjoyed during festivals and family gatherings, where crispy cutlets are paired with creamy potatoes, tangy kraut, or a squeeze of lemon. Fun fact: "schnitzel" comes from the German word Schnitt, meaning "slice."

INGREDIENTS:
- 2 boneless pork cutlets, pounded thin (about 100g each)
- ¼ cup flour
- 1 egg, beaten
- ½ cup breadcrumbs
- Salt and pepper, to taste
- 2 tbsp oil for frying
- 1 lemon, cut into wedges
- 2 cups arugula or mixed greens
- 1 tsp olive oil (for salad)

INSTRUCTIONS:

1. Season pork with salt and pepper. Dredge in flour, dip in egg, and coat in breadcrumbs.
2. Heat oil in a skillet over medium-high heat. Fry cutlets 3–4 minutes per side until crisp and golden.
3. Toss greens lightly in olive oil and plate with schnitzel.
4. Serve with lemon wedges for squeezing.

NUTRITION ESTIMATES (PER SERVING):
Calories: 520 | Protein: 35g | Carbs: 25g | Fat: 30g | Fiber: 2g

QUICK & EASY TIP: *Pound pork thin ahead of time or buy pre-cut schnitzel to save prep time.*

74. Quick Hungarian Goulash

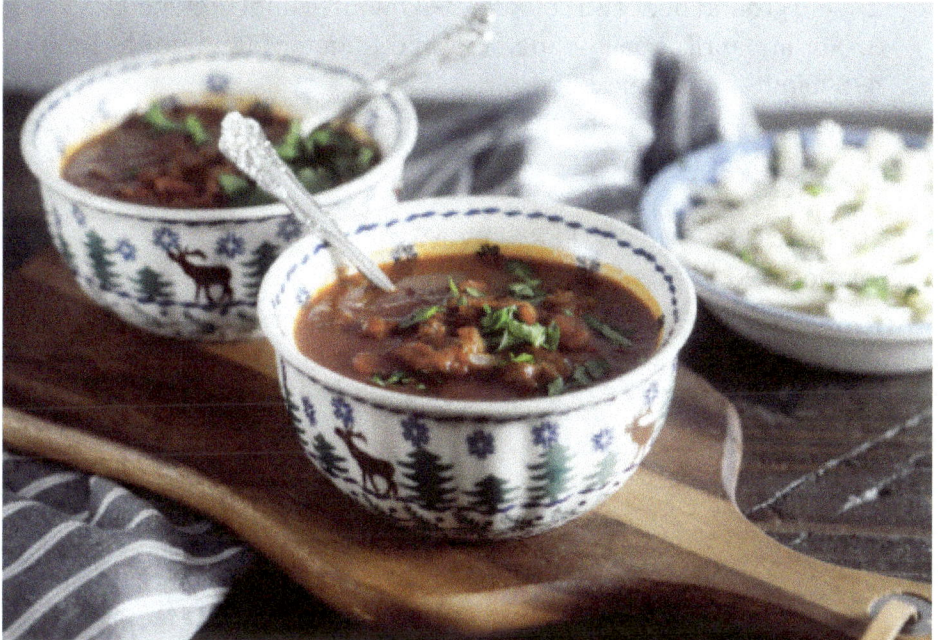

Prep Time: 5 minutes | Cook Time: 10 minutes | Makes: 2

Hungarian goulash (gulyás) is a national treasure, rooted in the traditions of 9th-century shepherds who slow-cooked beef in heavy cauldrons. Traditionally simmered for hours, the dish evolved from a rustic stew into a spiced comfort food found in homes and taverns across Hungary. This shortcut version captures the essence of goulash using tender ground beef, paprika, and peppers — all in just 15 minutes.

INGREDIENTS:
- 200g lean ground beef
- 1 tbsp olive oil
- 1 small onion, chopped
- 1 garlic clove, minced
- 1 tsp sweet Hungarian paprika (plus a pinch of smoked paprika, optional)
- ½ red bell pepper, chopped
- ½ cup crushed tomatoes
- ¼ cup beef broth or water
- Salt and black pepper, to taste
- Chopped parsley or sour cream, to garnish

INSTRUCTIONS:

1. Heat olive oil in a skillet over medium heat. Sauté onion and garlic for 1–2 minutes until soft.
2. Add ground beef and cook for 3–4 minutes until browned.
3. Stir in paprika, bell pepper, crushed tomatoes, and broth. Simmer for 4–5 minutes until thickened.
4. Season with salt and pepper. Serve hot, topped with parsley or a dollop of sour cream.

NUTRITION ESTIMATES (PER SERVING):
Calories: 390 | Protein: 27g | Carbs: 14g | Fat: 24g | Fiber: 3g

QUICK & EASY TIP: Use pre-chopped onions and garlic, and store-bought broth or tomato purée to keep prep under 5 minutes.

75. French Ratatouille Stir-Fry

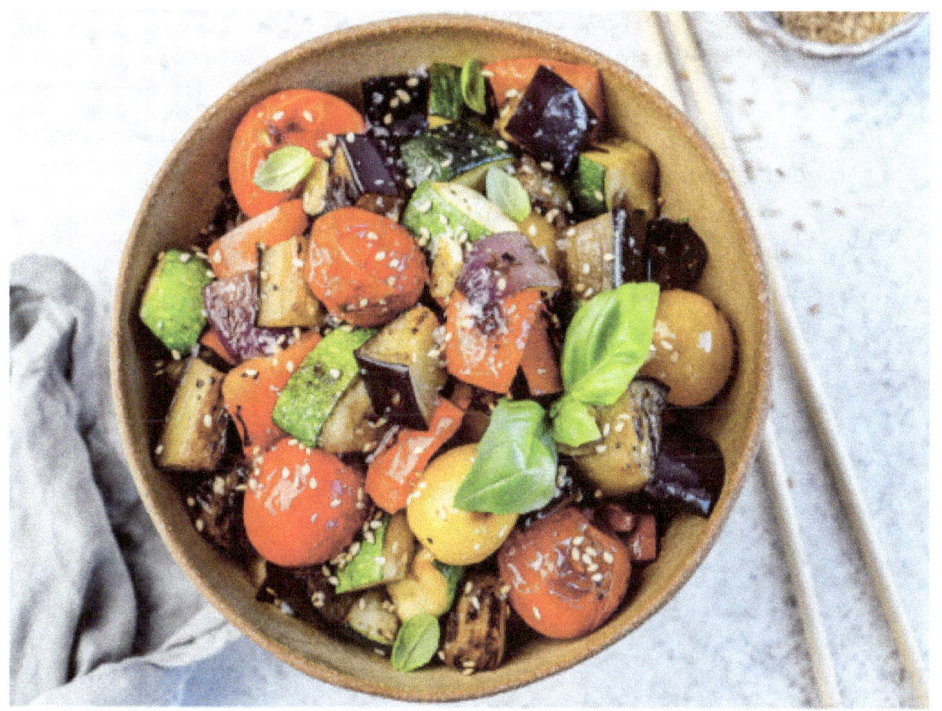

Prep Time: 4 minutes | Cook Time: 10 minutes | Makes: 2

This simplified take on French Ratatouille transforms the traditional slow-roasted vegetable medley into a speedy stir-fry packed with Mediterranean flavor—perfect with crusty bread or quinoa.

INGREDIENTS:
- ½ zucchini, chopped
- ½ eggplant, chopped
- ½ red bell pepper, chopped
- 1 small tomato, chopped
- 1 clove garlic, minced
- 1 tbsp olive oil
- ½ tsp dried herbes de Provence or Italian seasoning
- Salt and pepper, to taste
- Fresh basil or parsley, for garnish

INSTRUCTIONS:
1. Heat oil in a skillet. Sauté garlic and all veggies over high heat for 7–8 minutes until tender-crisp.
2. Add herbs, salt, and pepper. Stir well and cook for 1 more minute.

3. Garnish with fresh herbs and serve warm.

NUTRITION ESTIMATES (PER SERVING):
Calories: 180 | Protein: 4g | Carbs: 16g | Fat: 12g | Fiber: 5g

<u>QUICK & EASY TIP:</u> *Chop vegetables in advance and store refrigerated in a sealed container for up to 2 days.*

VIETNAMESE DINNERS

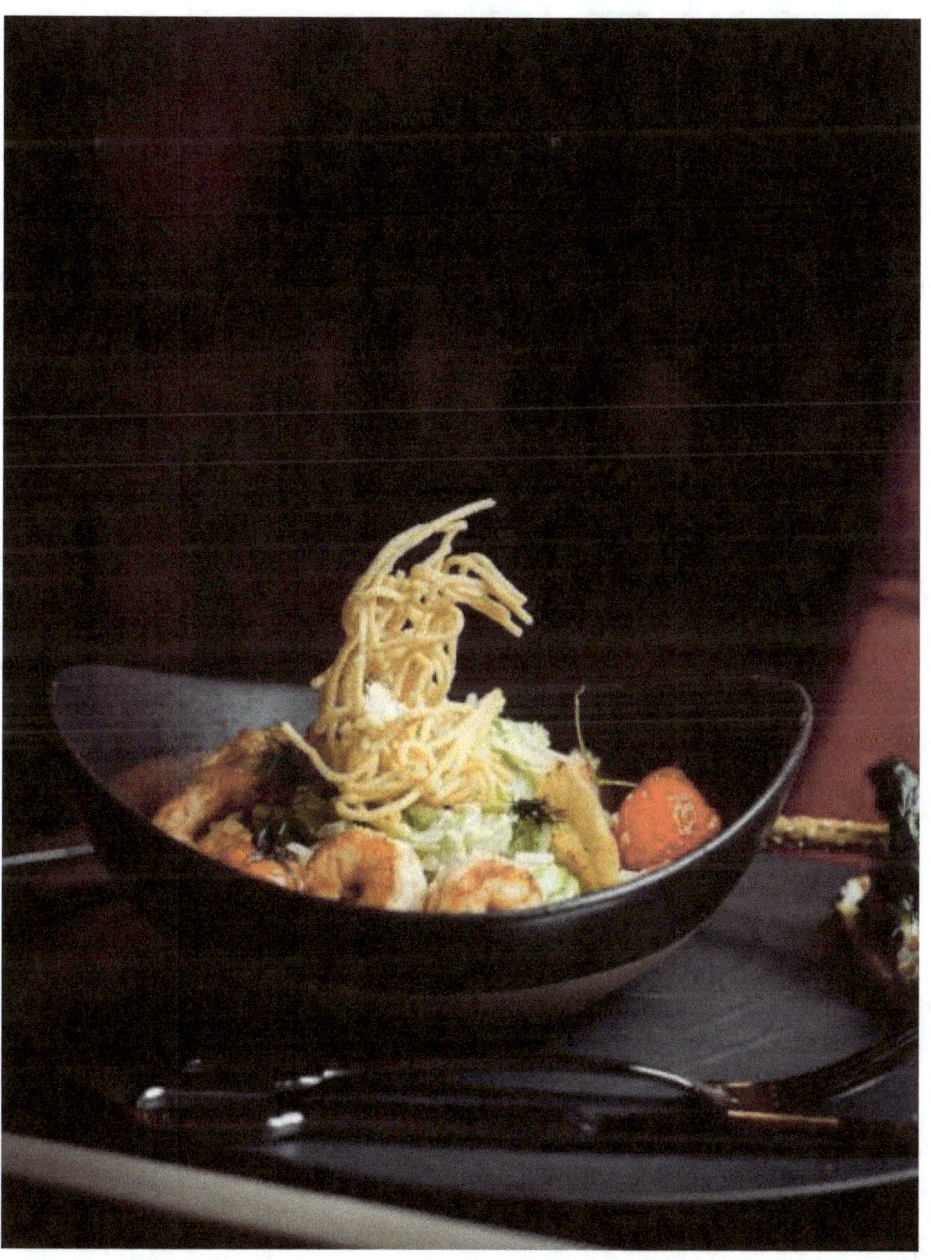

76. Vietnamese Shaking Beef

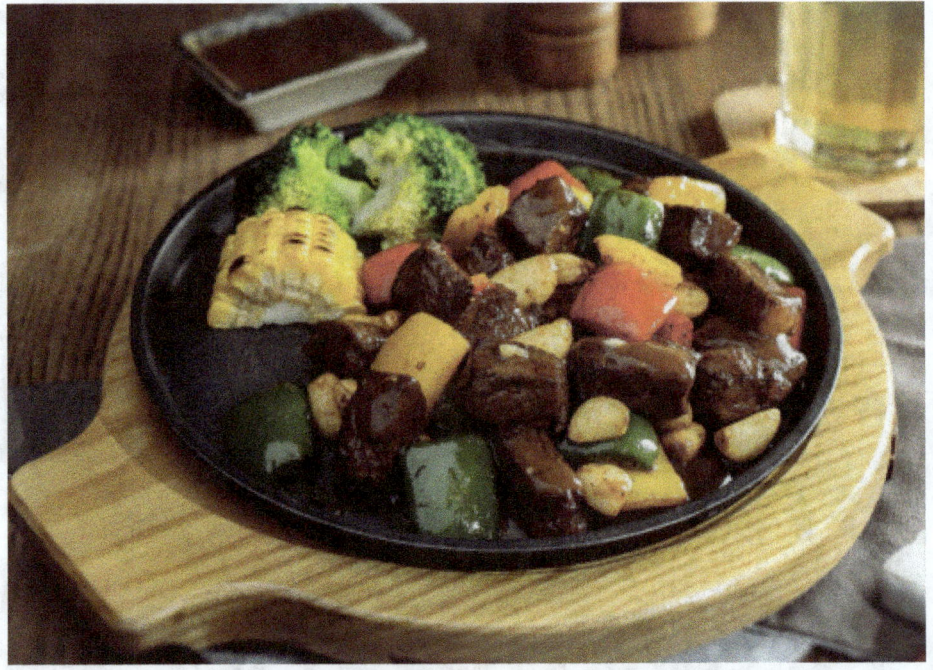

Prep Time: 5 minutes | Cook Time: 10 minutes | Makes: 2

Bò Lúc Lắc, or "shaking beef," gets its name from the quick searing and tossing of beef cubes in a hot pan. Originating during French colonial influence in Vietnam, it's a fusion of tender meat, savory-sweet marinade, and bright vegetables — a beloved dinner dish now served everywhere from street stalls to high-end restaurants.

INGREDIENTS:
- 200g sirloin or tenderloin, cut into 1-inch cubes
- 1 tbsp soy sauce
- 1 tsp oyster sauce
- 1 tsp sugar
- 1 tsp fish sauce
- 1 garlic clove, minced
- 1 tbsp oil
- ½ red onion, sliced
- 1 cup lettuce or watercress
- ½ cucumber, sliced
- Lime wedges and black pepper, to serve

INSTRUCTIONS:

1. Marinate beef in soy sauce, oyster sauce, sugar, fish sauce, and garlic. Let sit while you prep vegetables.
2. Heat oil in a large pan over high heat. Add beef and sear 3–4 minutes, shaking the pan often to brown all sides.
3. Add red onion and cook another 1–2 minutes.
4. Serve hot over lettuce and cucumber with lime and cracked pepper.

NUTRITION ESTIMATES (PER SERVING):
Calories: 450 | Protein: 34g | Carbs: 10g | Fat: 30g | Fiber: 2g

QUICK & EASY TIP: Use pre-cut beef stir-fry strips and marinate earlier in the day to cut active time.

77. Vietnamese Lemongrass Chicken

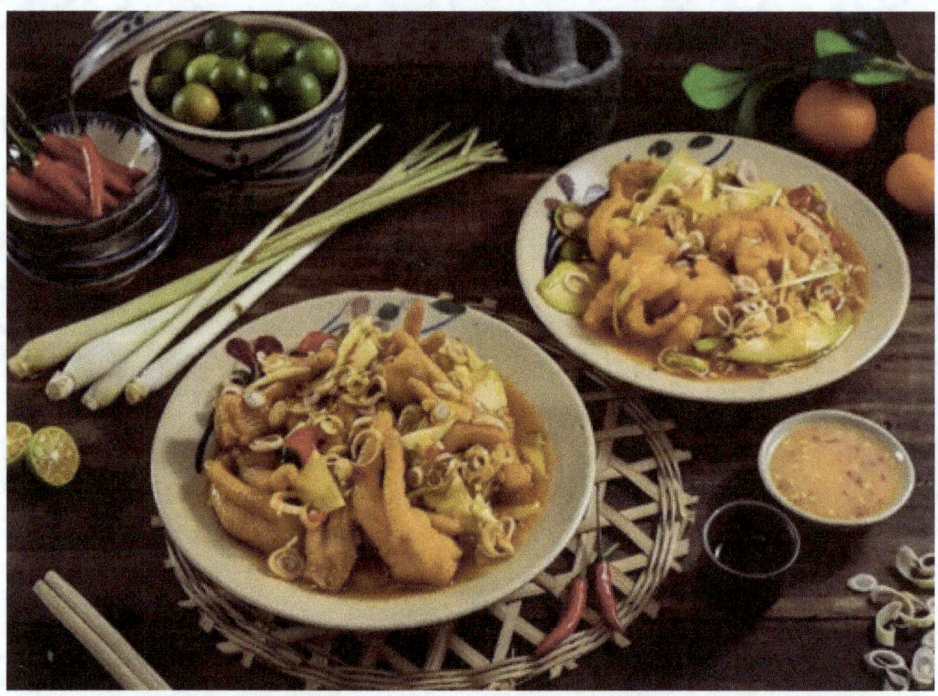

Prep Time: 5 minutes | Cook Time: 10 minutes | Makes: 2

Gà Xào Sả Ớt is a staple in southern Vietnamese kitchens, known for its bold flavors and intoxicating aroma. Lemongrass, a cornerstone of Vietnamese cuisine, brings a citrusy kick that pairs beautifully with chili heat. Traditionally cooked in well-worn woks over open flames, this quick stir-fry version delivers all the signature flair — spicy, savory, and deeply fragrant — in just minutes.

INGREDIENTS:
- 200g boneless chicken thighs, sliced thin
- 1 stalk lemongrass (white part only), minced (or 1 tbsp pre-minced)
- 1 garlic clove, minced
- 1 small red chili, sliced (optional)
- 1 tbsp fish sauce
- 1 tsp soy sauce
- ½ tsp sugar
- 1 tbsp oil
- Cooked jasmine rice, to serve
- Optional: chopped green onion or cilantro

INSTRUCTIONS:

1. Heat oil in a skillet or wok over medium heat. Add garlic, lemongrass, and chili. Sauté 1–2 minutes until fragrant.
2. Add chicken, fish sauce, soy sauce, and sugar. Stir-fry 6–8 minutes until chicken is browned and cooked through.
3. Garnish and serve hot over rice.

NUTRITION ESTIMATES (PER SERVING):
Calories: 460 | Protein: 32g | Carbs: 25g | Fat: 26g | Fiber: 1g

QUICK & EASY TIP: *Use pre-minced lemongrass or lemongrass paste to skip chopping.*

78. Vietnamese Skillet Egg Meatloaf

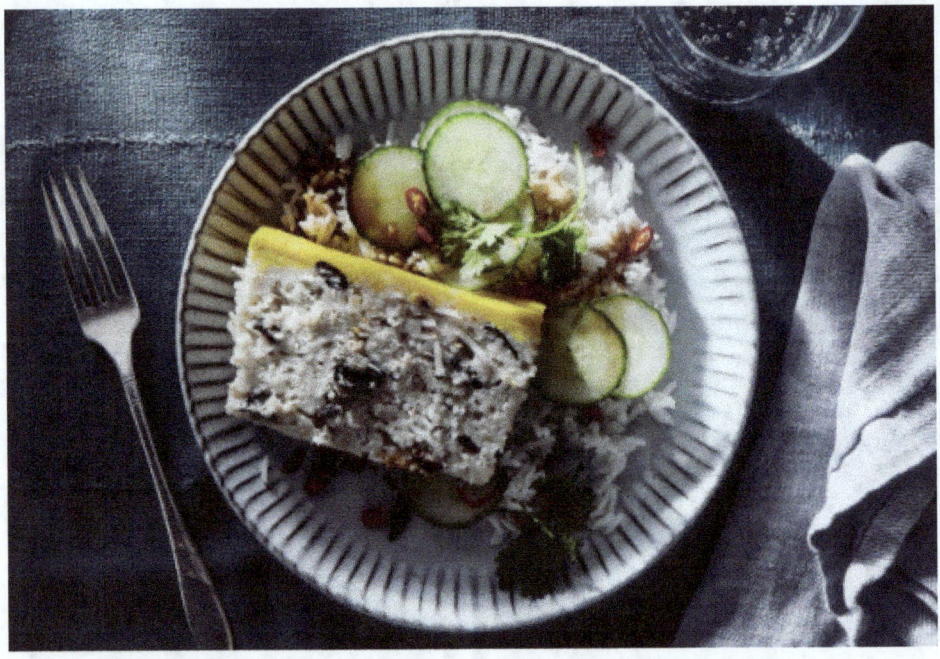

Prep Time: 5 minutes | Cook Time: 10 minutes | Makes: 2

Chả Trứng Hấp is a comforting Vietnamese classic often found in home-cooked meals and lunchbox spreads. This savory egg meatloaf, typically steamed over rice, combines ground meat, fish sauce, and eggs into a light yet hearty dish. Our stovetop version mimics the soft, custardy texture of the original in a fraction of the time—perfect for busy nights without sacrificing tradition.

INGREDIENTS:
- 200g ground pork or chicken
- 2 eggs
- 1 garlic clove, minced
- 1 tbsp fish sauce
- 1 tsp sugar
- ¼ small onion, minced
- Pinch of pepper
- Chopped green onions (optional)

INSTRUCTIONS:

1. In a bowl, mix ground meat, 1 egg, garlic, onion, fish sauce, sugar, and pepper.
2. Spread mixture into a lightly oiled small skillet. Cover and cook over medium heat for 6–7 minutes.
3. Beat the second egg and pour over the top. Cover and cook 2–3 more minutes until set.
4. Slice and serve with hot rice.

NUTRITION ESTIMATES (PER SERVING):
Calories: 410 | Protein: 30g | Carbs: 4g | Fat: 28g | Fiber: 0g

QUICK & EASY TIP: Use a nonstick pan with a lid for quick "steaming" on the stovetop.

| 79. | Beef and Water Spinach Stir-Fry |

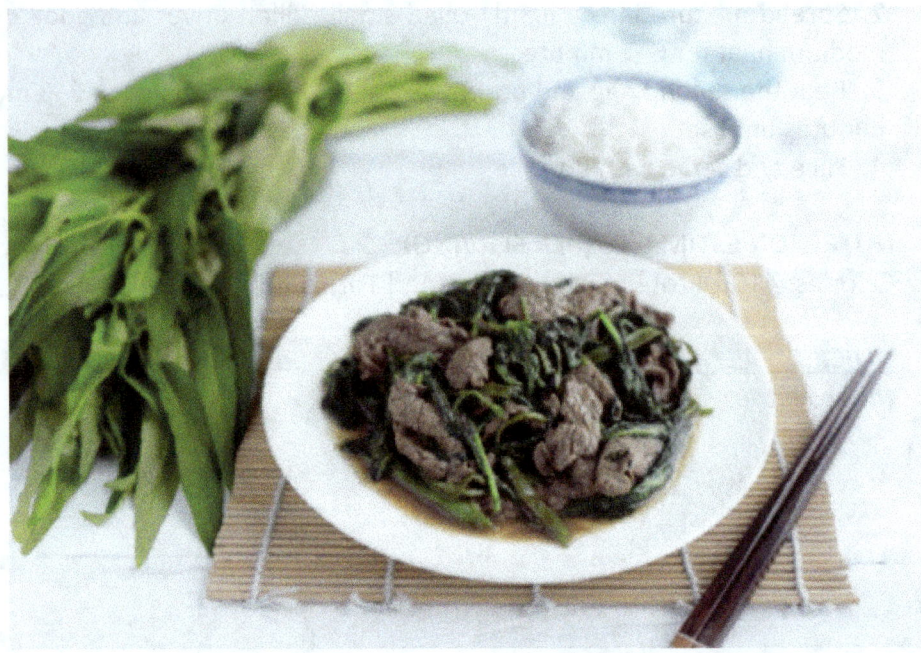

Prep Time: 5 minutes | Cook Time: 10 minutes | Makes: 2

In Vietnam, rau muống xào thịt bò is a beloved home-style stir-fry found everywhere from countryside kitchens to city cafés. Water spinach (rau muống), known for its crunchy hollow stems and tender leaves, is a staple of Vietnamese cuisine and often harvested fresh from riverside farms. Stir-fried quickly with beef and garlic, this dish is all about balance—light, savory, and full of texture, it's a true taste of everyday Vietnam.

INGREDIENTS:
- 200g beef (sirloin or flank), thinly sliced
- 150g water spinach (or substitute with baby spinach or bok choy)
- 2 garlic cloves, minced
- 1 tbsp oyster sauce
- 1 tsp soy sauce
- ½ tsp sugar
- 1 tbsp oil
- Cooked jasmine rice, to serve

INSTRUCTIONS:
1. Heat oil in a large pan or wok. Sauté garlic for 30 seconds.
2. Add beef, oyster sauce, soy sauce, and sugar. Stir-fry for 3–4 minutes until just browned.

3. Add water spinach and stir-fry 1–2 more minutes until wilted but still vibrant.
4. Serve hot with rice.

NUTRITION ESTIMATES (PER SERVING):
Calories: 440 | Protein: 33g | Carbs: 22g | Fat: 25g | Fiber: 3g

<u>*QUICK & EASY TIP:*</u> *Pre-sliced beef and pre-washed greens reduce total time significantly.*

80. Vietnamese Tamarind Shrimp

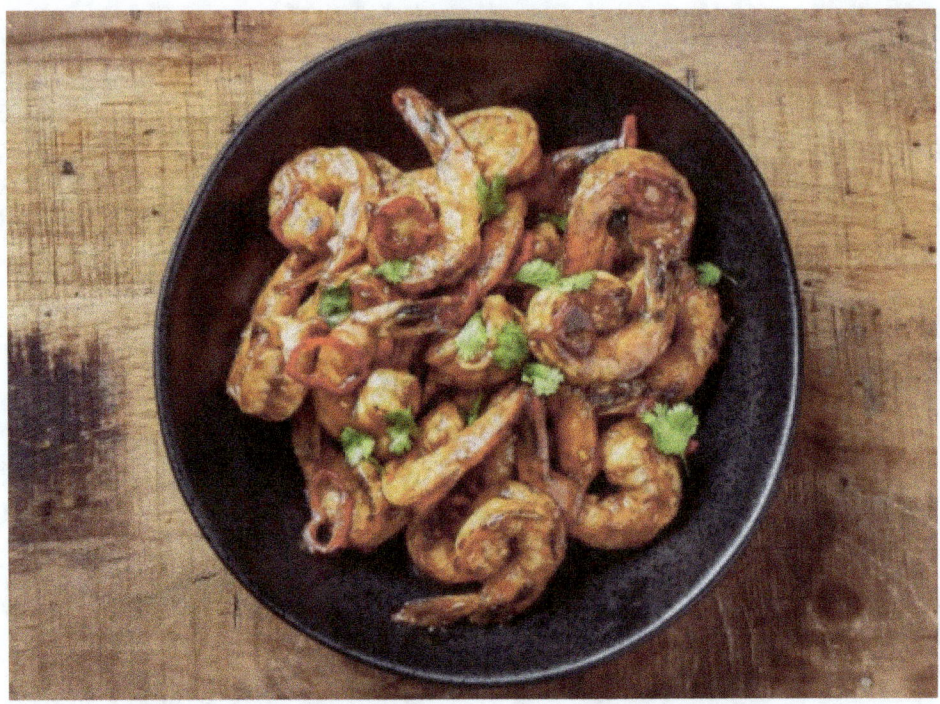

Prep Time: 5 minutes | Cook Time: 10 minutes | Makes: 2

This sweet-sour-spicy dish features shrimp simmered in tamarind sauce — a beloved coastal dinner from southern Vietnam. Traditionally slow-cooked, this shortcut version uses ready-made tamarind paste and quick sautéeing for full flavor fast.

INGREDIENTS:
- 200g peeled shrimp
- 1 tbsp tamarind paste (or 1 tsp tamarind concentrate + 2 tbsp water)
- 1 tsp fish sauce
- 1 tsp sugar
- 1 garlic clove, minced
- 1 tbsp oil
- Chili slices or flakes (optional)
- Cooked rice, to serve

INSTRUCTIONS:
1. Mix tamarind paste, fish sauce, and sugar in a bowl.
2. Heat oil in a skillet. Sauté garlic for 1 minute, then add shrimp.
3. Pour in tamarind mixture. Cook 4–5 minutes until shrimp are pink and sauce thickens.

4. Add chili if using, and serve hot over rice.

NUTRITION ESTIMATES (PER SERVING):
Calories: 390 | Protein: 30g | Carbs: 16g | Fat: 22g | Fiber: 1g

QUICK & EASY TIP: Use deveined, peeled shrimp and premixed sauce to save at least 5 minutes of prep.

CHINESE DINNERS

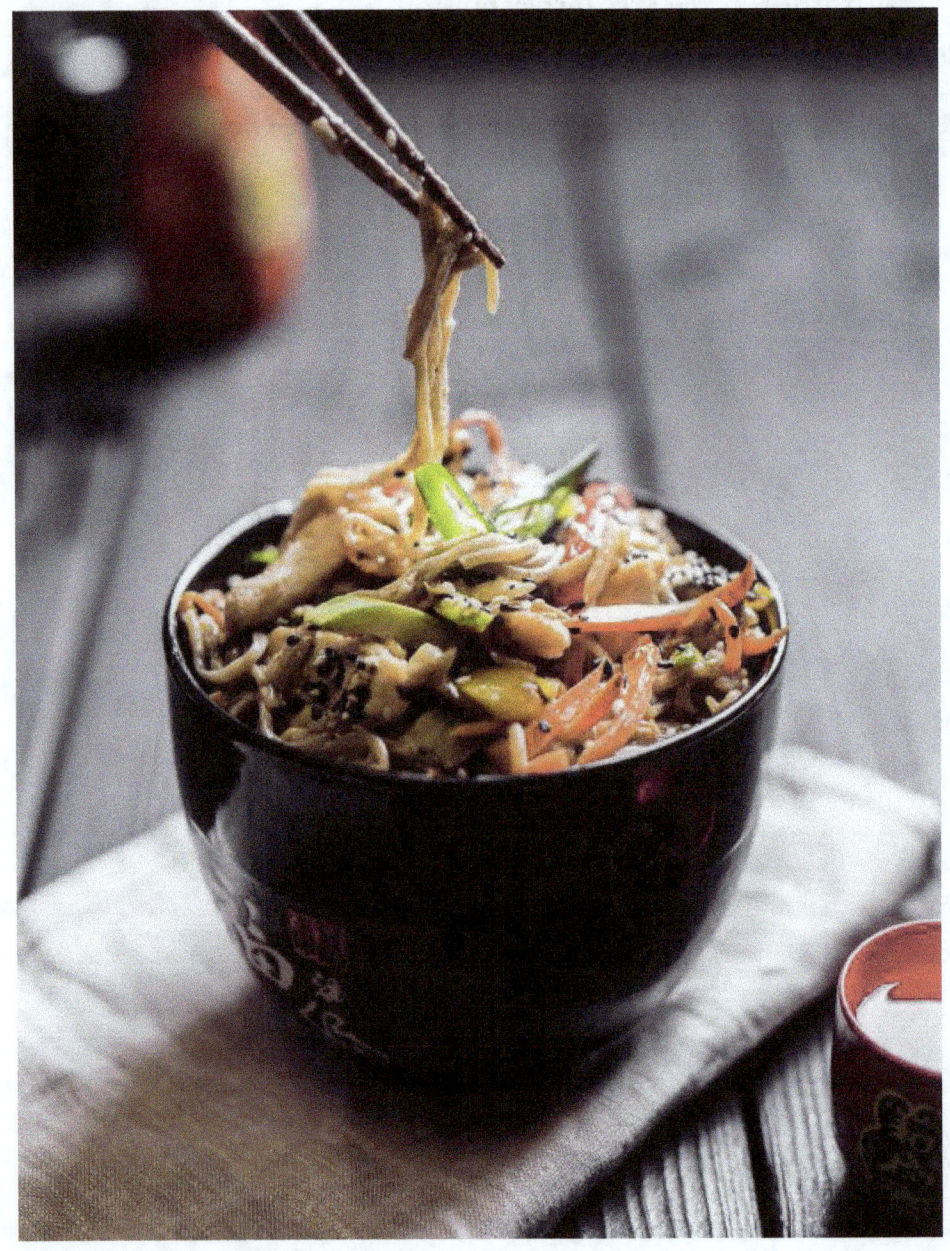

81. Chicken Manchurian

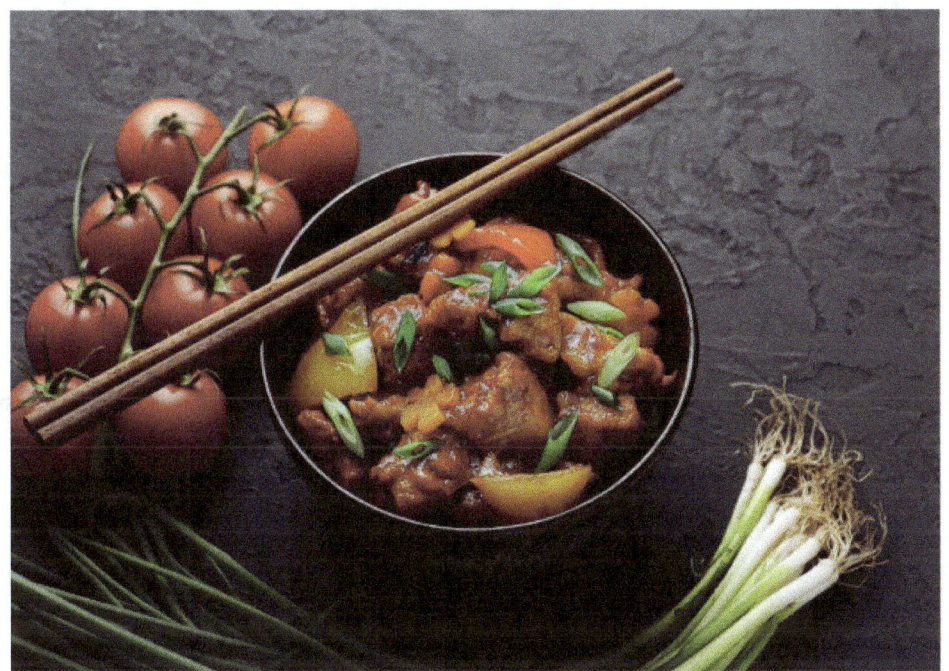

Prep Time: 5 minutes | Cook Time: 9 minutes | Makes: 2

Chicken Manchurian is a beloved Indo-Chinese fusion dish featuring crispy chicken tossed in a tangy, spicy soy-based sauce. Though usually deep-fried, this quick version pan-fries the chicken to cut down on time without sacrificing texture or flavor.

INGREDIENTS:
- 250g boneless chicken, cubed
- 2 tbsp cornstarch
- 1 tbsp all-purpose flour
- Salt and pepper, to taste
- 1 tbsp oil
- 1 tsp ginger-garlic paste
- 2 tbsp chopped onion
- 2 tbsp chopped bell pepper
- 2 tbsp soy sauce
- 1 tbsp ketchup
- 1 tsp chili sauce (optional)
- ¼ cup water
- 1 tsp cornstarch (mixed with 1 tbsp water)
- Chopped spring onions, for garnish

INSTRUCTIONS:
1. Toss chicken with cornstarch, flour, salt, and pepper. Pan-fry in oil until lightly golden. Remove and set aside.
2. In the same pan, sauté onion, bell pepper, and ginger-garlic paste for 2 minutes.
3. Add sauces and ¼ cup water. Stir in cornstarch slurry to thicken.
4. Add chicken back in and toss to coat. Garnish with spring onions.

NUTRITION ESTIMATES (PER SERVING):
Calories: 380 | Protein: 30g | Carbs: 16g | Fat: 22g | Fiber: 2g

<u>QUICK & EASY TIP:</u> Use thin chicken cubes and a nonstick pan for faster searing. Sauce base can be pre-mixed and refrigerated for later.

82. Beef and Mushroom Noodles with Broth

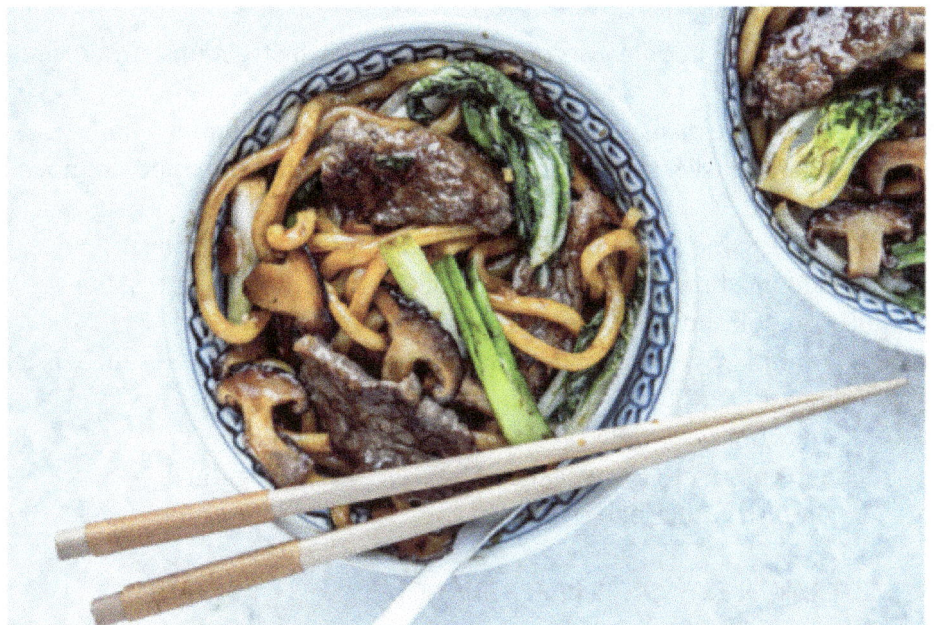

Prep Time: 15 minutes | Cook Time: 15 minutes | Makes: 4 servings

This hearty noodle bowl is inspired by Chinese-style beef noodle soups, popular across East Asia for their deeply comforting flavors. Though traditionally simmered for hours, this version delivers rich, umami-packed broth in minutes. The combination of mushrooms, bok choy, and tender beef captures the soul of a warming street-side noodle dish without the wait.

INGREDIENTS:
- 1 lb (450 g) beef sirloin or flank steak, thinly sliced
- 8 oz (225 g) whole wheat or rice noodles
- 2 tablespoons olive oil
- 1 cup mushrooms, sliced
- 1 red bell pepper, thinly sliced
- 2 cups bok choy, chopped
- 2 cloves garlic, minced
- 1 tablespoon fresh ginger, minced
- 4 cups bone broth
- 2 tablespoons soy sauce
- 1 tablespoon rice vinegar
- 1 tablespoon hoisin sauce (optional)
- 2 green onions, sliced

- 1 tablespoon sesame seeds (optional)

INSTRUCTIONS:
1. Cook the noodles according to package instructions. Drain and set aside.
2. Heat olive oil in a large skillet or wok over medium-high heat.
3. Add beef slices and cook for 4–5 minutes until browned. Remove and set aside.
4. In the same skillet, sauté garlic and ginger for 30 seconds.
5. Add mushrooms and bell pepper. Stir-fry for 3–4 minutes.
6. Add bok choy and cook for 2 minutes until wilted.
7. Pour in bone broth, soy sauce, rice vinegar, and hoisin sauce. Bring to a simmer.
8. Add cooked noodles and toss to heat through.
9. Return beef to the skillet and mix everything together.
10. Garnish with green onions and sesame seeds if desired.

NUTRITION ESTIMATES (PER SERVING):
Calories: 350 | Protein: 25g | Carbohydrates: 35g | Fat: 12g | Fiber: 4g

<u>QUICK & EASY TIP:</u> For quicker prep, use pre-sliced stir-fry beef and ready-to-eat noodles found in the refrigerated section. Pre-chopped bok choy mix or frozen stir-fry vegetables also work great.

83. Beef and Broccoli Stir-Fry

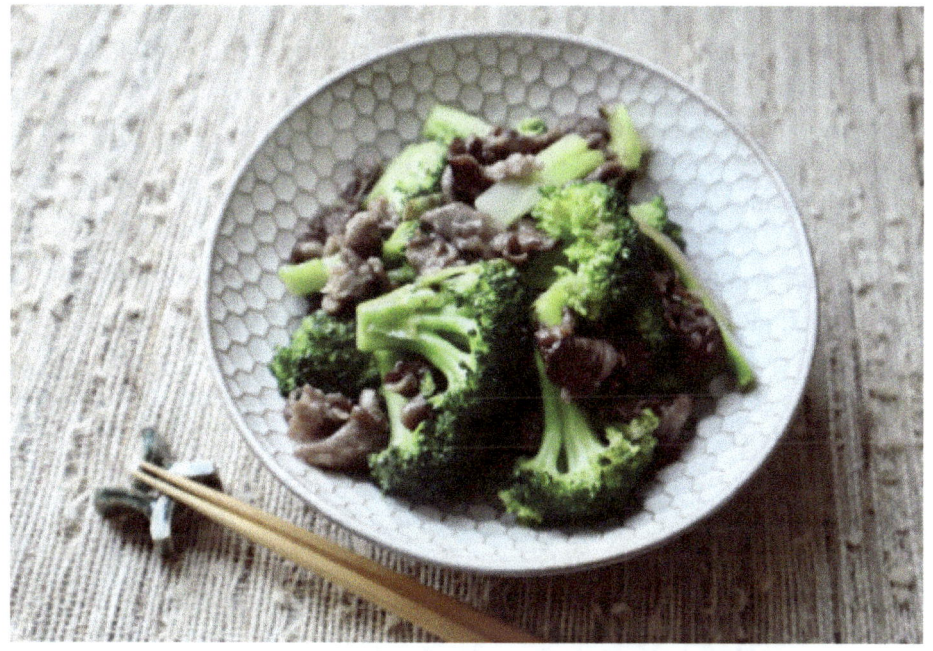

Prep Time: 5 minutes | Cook Time: 10 minutes | Makes: 2

Though popularized by Chinese-American restaurants, Beef and Broccoli is inspired by Cantonese stir-fry traditions. It swaps Chinese gai lan (Chinese broccoli) for the more widely available Western broccoli, creating a dish that's both comforting and adaptable. With tender beef, crisp vegetables, and a savory soy-based sauce, it's a quick, flavorful staple that reflects the evolution of Chinese cuisine abroad.

INGREDIENTS:
- 200g beef (flank or sirloin), thinly sliced
- 1½ cups broccoli florets
- 2 garlic cloves, minced
- 1 tbsp soy sauce
- 1 tsp oyster sauce
- 1 tsp cornstarch
- ½ tsp sugar
- 2 tbsp water
- 1 tbsp oil
- Cooked jasmine rice, to serve

INSTRUCTIONS:

1. Mix beef with soy sauce, oyster sauce, sugar, and cornstarch. Set aside.
2. Blanch broccoli in hot water or microwave for 2 minutes.
3. Heat oil in a wok. Stir-fry garlic for 30 seconds, add beef and cook 3–4 minutes.
4. Add broccoli and 2 tbsp water. Stir-fry 1–2 more minutes until everything is coated and heated through.
5. Serve hot over rice.

NUTRITION ESTIMATES (PER SERVING):
Calories: 480 | Protein: 35g | Carbs: 24g | Fat: 26g | Fiber: 3g

QUICK & EASY TIP: Use pre-sliced beef and microwave the broccoli to shave off prep time.

> **84.**   **Chinese Tomato and Egg Stir-Fry**

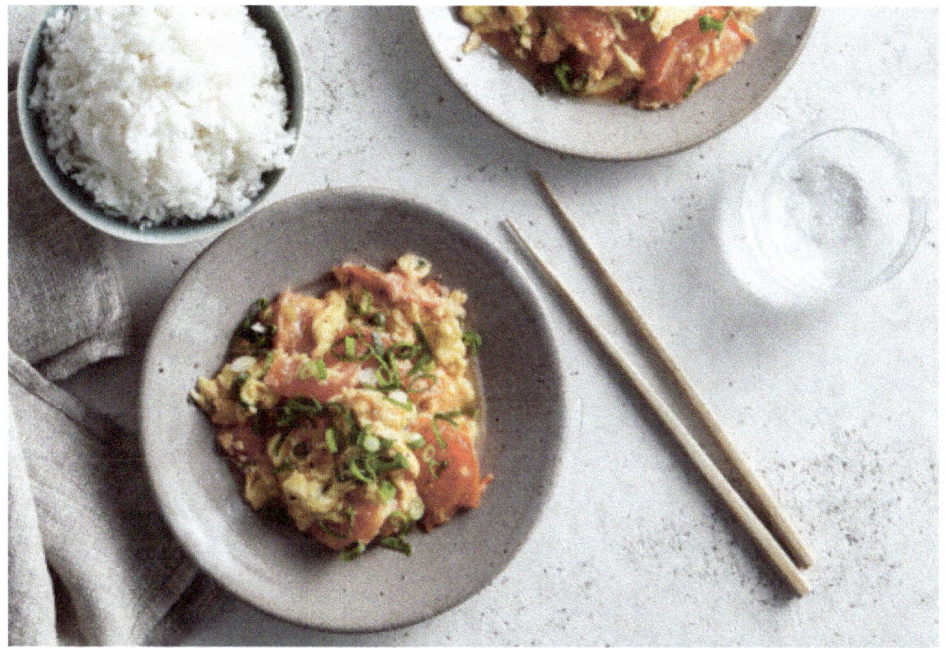

Prep Time: 3 minutes | Cook Time: 7 minutes | Makes: 2

A comfort-food staple across China, this dish combines soft-scrambled eggs with lightly stewed tomatoes — sweet, tangy, and satisfying. It's fast, nutritious, and often considered a go-to dinner for students, workers, and home cooks alike.

INGREDIENTS:
- 3 eggs
- 2 medium tomatoes, cut into wedges
- 1 garlic clove, minced
- ½ tsp sugar
- Salt, to taste
- 1 tbsp oil
- Chopped green onion (optional)
- Cooked rice, to serve

INSTRUCTIONS:
1. Beat eggs with a pinch of salt.
2. Heat half the oil in a wok or skillet. Scramble eggs softly, remove, and set aside.
3. Add remaining oil, garlic, and tomatoes. Cook 2–3 minutes until tomatoes soften.

4. Return eggs to pan. Add sugar and stir-fry for 1 minute until just combined.
5. Serve over rice, topped with green onions if using.

NUTRITION ESTIMATES (PER SERVING):
Calories: 360 | Protein: 16g | Carbs: 14g | Fat: 26g | Fiber: 2g

QUICK & EASY TIP: Use ripe tomatoes and cook eggs gently to avoid over-drying — it comes together fast.

85. Kung Pao Chicken

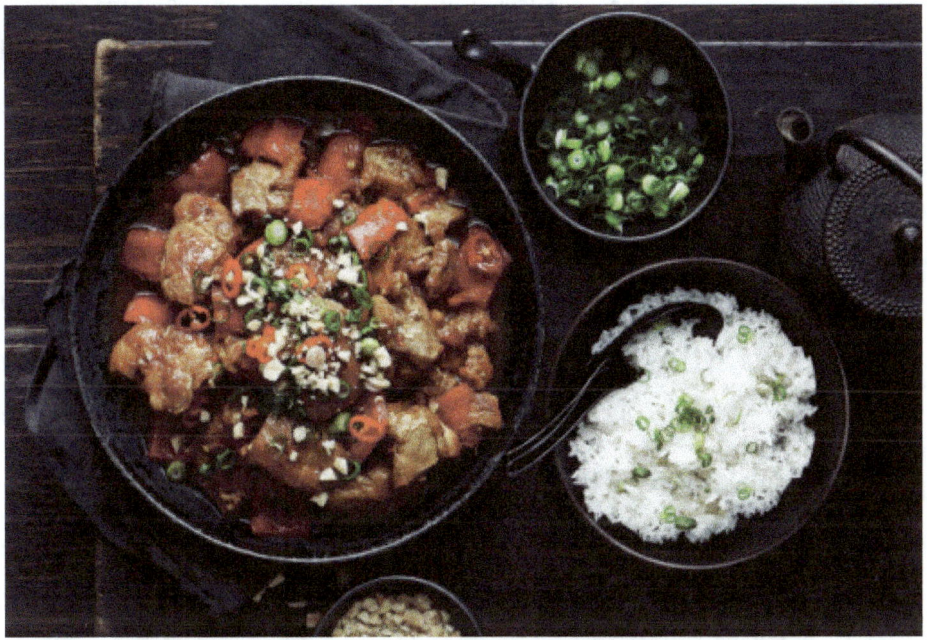

Prep Time: 5 minutes | Cook Time: 9 minutes | Makes: 2

Kung Pao Chicken (宫保鸡丁) hails from China's Sichuan province, famed for its fiery cuisine and use of numbing Sichuan peppercorns. Originally named after a Qing dynasty official, Ding Baozhen (a.k.a. "Kung Pao"), the dish has traveled far from its roots — now enjoyed in countless variations around the world. This quick take keeps the signature combo of tender chicken, chilies, and peanuts while using pantry shortcuts for maximum flavor in minimal time.

INGREDIENTS:
- 200g boneless chicken breast or thigh, diced
- 2 dried red chilies (optional)
- 2 garlic cloves, minced
- 1 tbsp soy sauce
- 1 tsp vinegar
- ½ tsp sugar
- ½ tsp cornstarch
- 1 tbsp oil
- 2 tbsp roasted peanuts
- 2 green onions, sliced
- Cooked rice, to serve

INSTRUCTIONS:
1. Mix chicken with soy sauce, sugar, and cornstarch.
2. Heat oil in a wok. Add dried chilies and garlic, stir-fry for 30 seconds.
3. Add chicken and cook 5–6 minutes until browned and cooked through.
4. Stir in vinegar, peanuts, and green onions. Cook 1–2 more minutes.
5. Serve hot over rice.

NUTRITION ESTIMATES (PER SERVING):
Calories: 470 | Protein: 34g | Carbs: 18g | Fat: 28g | Fiber: 2g

QUICK & EASY TIP: Use pre-diced chicken and roasted peanuts to save prep time.

86. Chinese Pepper Steak

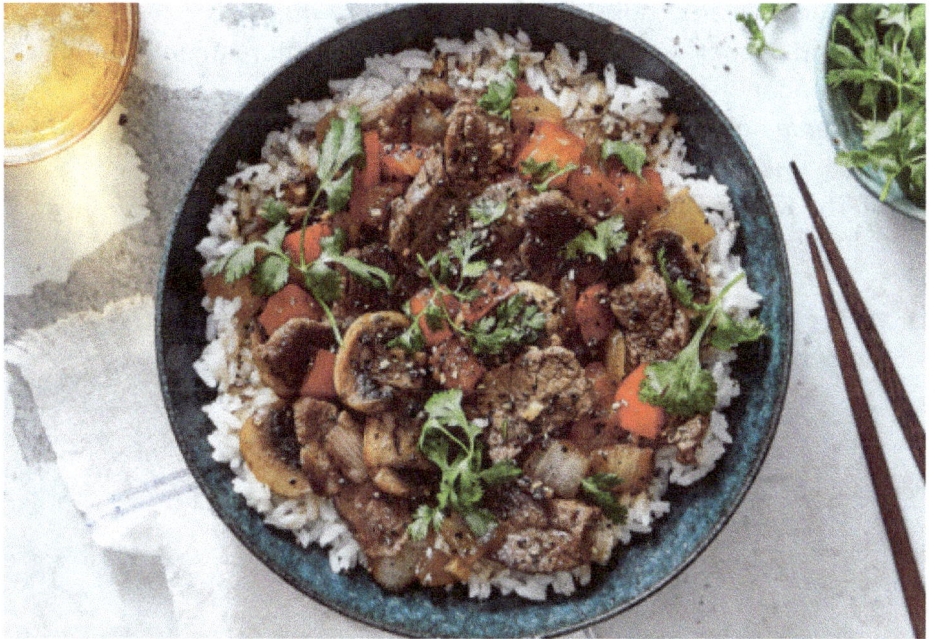

Prep Time: 5 minutes | Cook Time: 9 minutes | Makes: 2

While widely known through American Chinese restaurants, Pepper Steak has roots in Cantonese cuisine, where quick stir-frying preserves the crispness of vegetables and tenderness of meat. Its U.S. adaptation gained popularity in the mid-20th century as Chinese-American chefs blended traditional techniques with locally available ingredients like bell peppers and beef — a fun cultural fusion that continues to satisfy weeknight dinners today.

INGREDIENTS:
- 200g flank or sirloin steak, thinly sliced
- 1 small green bell pepper, sliced
- 1 small red bell pepper, sliced
- 1 garlic clove, minced
- 1 tbsp soy sauce
- 1 tsp oyster sauce
- ½ tsp sugar
- 1 tsp cornstarch
- 1 tbsp oil
- Cooked jasmine rice, to serve

INSTRUCTIONS:

1. Toss beef with soy sauce, sugar, and cornstarch.
2. Heat oil in a wok over high heat. Sauté garlic for 30 seconds.
3. Add beef and cook 2–3 minutes until browned.
4. Add peppers and oyster sauce. Stir-fry 3–4 more minutes until veggies are tender-crisp.
5. Serve hot over rice.

NUTRITION ESTIMATES (PER SERVING):
Calories: 480 | Protein: 34g | Carbs: 20g | Fat: 30g | Fiber: 3g

<u>*QUICK & EASY TIP:*</u> *Pre-slice beef and peppers earlier in the day or buy pre-cut stir-fry packs to save prep time.*

| 87. | Garlic Bok Choy with Tofu |

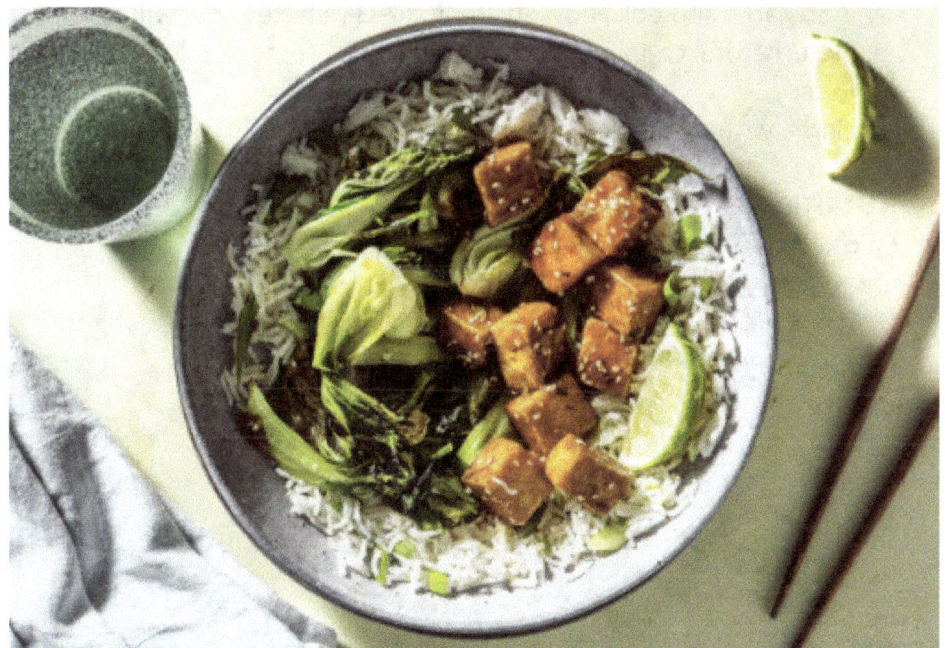

Prep Time: 4 minutes | Cook Time: 10 minutes | Makes: 2

A beloved dish in Chinese Buddhist cuisine, this stir-fry reflects the tradition of zhāi cài — vegetarian meals often eaten for spiritual or health reasons. Tofu and bok choy are pantry staples in many Chinese households, prized not just for their nutrition but for their balance of texture: tender-crisp greens and golden tofu cubes, all brought together with fragrant garlic.

INGREDIENTS:
- 200g firm tofu, cubed
- 150g baby bok choy, halved
- 2 garlic cloves, minced
- 1 tbsp soy sauce
- 1 tsp sesame oil
- 1 tbsp oil
- Salt, to taste
- Cooked rice, to serve

INSTRUCTIONS:

1. Heat oil in a pan. Pan-fry tofu cubes for 5 minutes until golden on all sides. Remove.
2. Add garlic and bok choy. Stir-fry for 2–3 minutes until wilted.
3. Return tofu to pan, add soy sauce and sesame oil. Stir-fry 1 more minute.
4. Serve with steamed rice.

NUTRITION ESTIMATES (PER SERVING):
Calories: 400 | Protein: 20g | Carbs: 15g | Fat: 28g | Fiber: 3g

<u>QUICK & EASY TIP:</u> Use pre-cubed tofu and pre-washed baby bok choy for maximum speed.

88. Tofu and Mushroom Stir-Fry

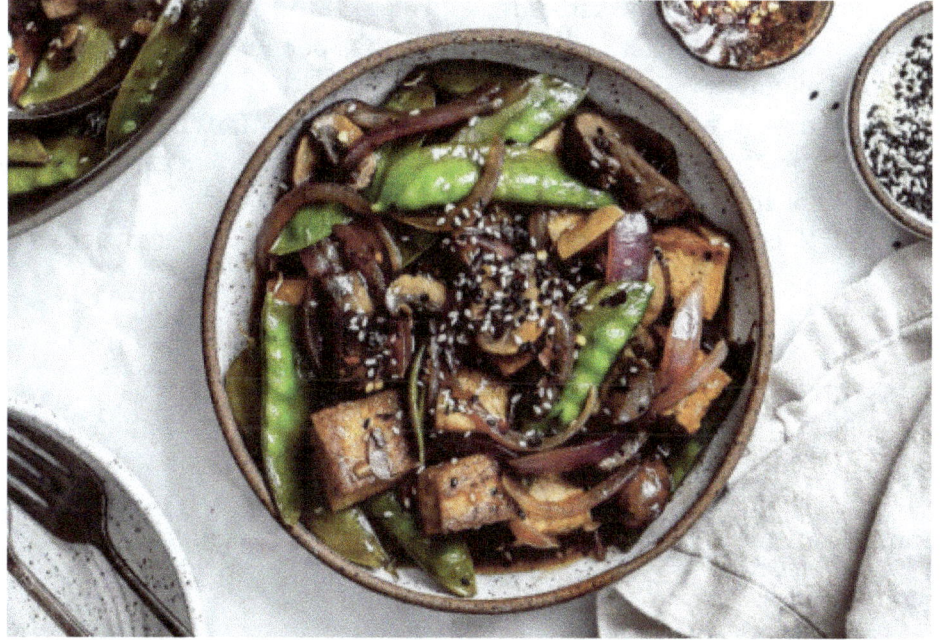

Prep Time: 10 min | Cook Time: 15 min | Makes: 4 servings

Rooted in traditional Chinese vegetarian cooking, tofu and mushroom stir-fries are especially common in Buddhist temples, where meatless meals emphasize balance, texture, and umami-rich flavors. This modern version keeps those principles alive — combining tender tofu and earthy mushrooms for a comforting dish now embraced across global kitchens.

INGREDIENTS:
- 1 block firm tofu, drained and cubed
- 2 tablespoons olive oil
- 1 cup mushrooms, sliced
- 1 red bell pepper, sliced
- 1 cup snap peas
- 2 cloves garlic, minced
- 1 tablespoon ginger, minced
- 3 tablespoons soy sauce
- 1 tablespoon rice vinegar
- 1 teaspoon sesame oil
- 1 tablespoon cornstarch mixed with 2 tablespoons water (optional, for thickening)

INSTRUCTIONS:

1. Heat olive oil in a large skillet or wok over medium-high heat.
2. Add tofu cubes and cook until golden brown on all sides, about 7–8 minutes. Remove and set aside.
3. In the same skillet, add mushrooms, bell pepper, and snap peas. Cook for 5 minutes.
4. Add garlic and ginger. Cook for another 1–2 minutes until fragrant.
5. Return tofu to the skillet. Stir in soy sauce, rice vinegar, and sesame oil. Cook for 2 more minutes.
6. If thicker sauce is desired, add cornstarch slurry and cook for 1 minute.
7. Serve warm.

NUTRITION ESTIMATES (PER SERVING):
Calories: 180 | Protein: 12g | Carbohydrates: 15g | Fat: 9g | Fiber: 4g

QUICK & EASY TIP: Save time by using pre-cubed tofu and frozen stir-fry vegetable blends from the store.

| 89. | Ginger Sesame Chicken Stir-Fry |

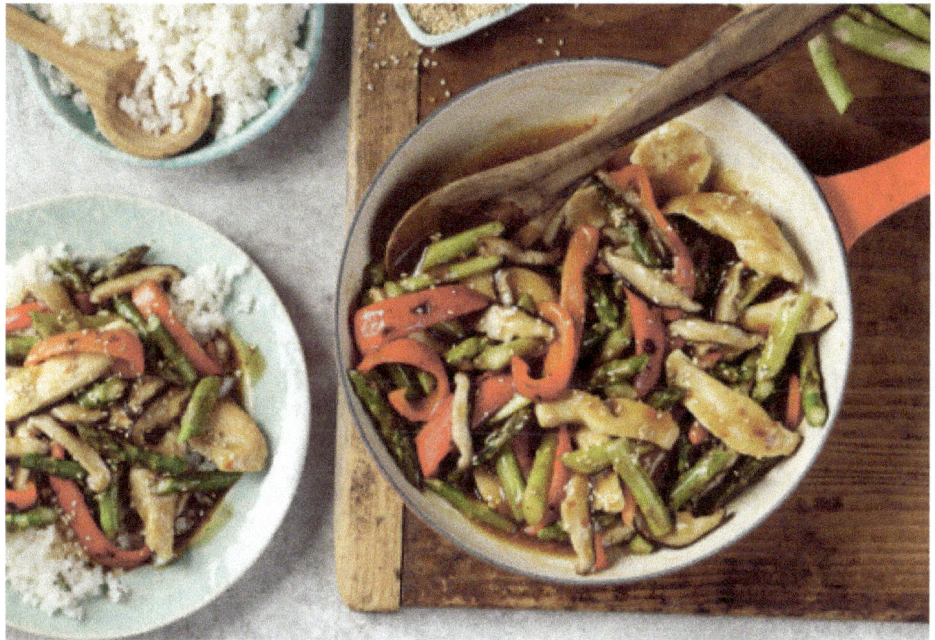

Prep Time: 15 min | Cook Time: 15 min | Makes: 4 servings

Quick stir-fries like this are the heartbeat of weeknight Chinese meals. With its gingery aroma, crisp vegetables, and nutty sesame oil, this dish reflects the core of Chinese wok cooking—simple ingredients cooked fast over high heat to preserve texture and flavor.

INGREDIENTS:
- 1 lb (450 g) boneless, skinless chicken breast, thinly sliced
- 2 tbsp sesame oil
- 1 cup bell peppers, sliced
- 1 cup carrots, julienned
- 1 cup green beans, trimmed
- 1 tbsp fresh ginger, minced
- 2 tbsp tamari (gluten-free soy sauce)
- 1 tbsp rice vinegar
- 1 tsp sesame seeds
- Salt and pepper to taste

INSTRUCTIONS:
1. Heat sesame oil in a wok or large pan over medium-high heat.
2. Add chicken and cook for 5–7 minutes until fully cooked. Remove and set aside.

3. Add bell peppers, carrots, and green beans. Stir-fry for 4–5 minutes.
4. Add minced ginger and cook for 1 minute.
5. Return chicken to the pan. Stir in tamari and vinegar. Cook 2–3 minutes.
6. Garnish with sesame seeds and serve.

NUTRITION ESTIMATES (PER SERVING):
Calories: 280 | Protein: 30g | Carbohydrates: 15g | Fat: 14g | Fiber: 3g

QUICK & EASY TIP: *Use pre-sliced chicken breast and frozen vegetable stir-fry mix to reduce prep time.*

90. Salmon Fried Rice

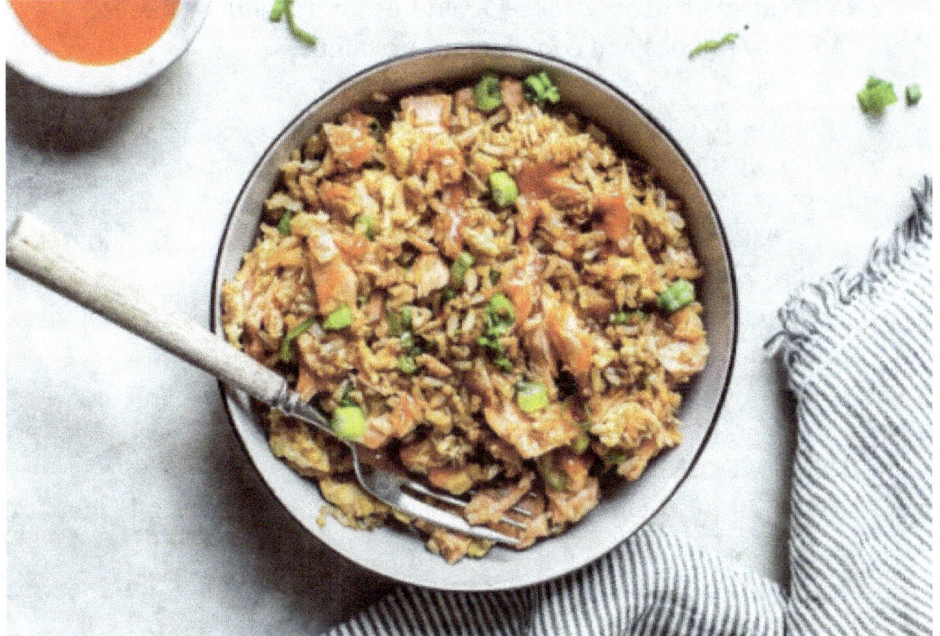

Prep Time: 10 min | Cook Time: 15 min | Makes: 4 servings

Fried rice dates back to the Sui Dynasty in China as a practical way to repurpose day-old rice and leftover ingredients — nothing went to waste. This modern twist features flaked salmon, adding a boost of protein and omega-3s to the traditional dish. It's fast, satisfying, and a perfect example of how Chinese culinary ingenuity adapts across time and cultures.

INGREDIENTS:
- 2 cups cooked white or jasmine rice (preferably cold and day-old for best texture)
- 1 tbsp olive oil
- 1 cup cooked salmon, flaked (use leftover or pre-cooked salmon)
- ½ cup diced carrots
- ½ cup frozen peas
- 2 large eggs, lightly beaten
- 2 green onions, chopped
- 2 tbsp gluten-free soy sauce
- ½ tsp sesame oil (optional)
- Salt and pepper to taste
- 1 tbsp chopped fresh cilantro (for garnish, optional)

INSTRUCTIONS:
1. Heat olive oil in a large skillet or wok over medium heat.
2. Add carrots and cook for 3–4 minutes until slightly softened.
3. Add frozen peas and cook for 2 more minutes.
4. Push vegetables to one side. Add beaten eggs to the other side and scramble until fully cooked. Mix with vegetables.
5. Add cold rice, breaking up clumps. Stir to combine with vegetables and eggs.
6. Add flaked salmon and green onions. Cook for 2–3 minutes until heated through.
7. Pour in soy sauce and sesame oil (if using). Stir to evenly coat.
8. Season with salt and pepper.
9. Garnish with cilantro if desired and serve hot.

NUTRITION ESTIMATES (PER SERVING):
Calories: 320 | Protein: 18g | Carbohydrates: 35g | Fat: 12g | Fiber: 2g

QUICK & EASY TIP: *Use microwave-ready rice and canned or pre-cooked salmon to cut prep time by half.*

MALAYSIAN DINNERS

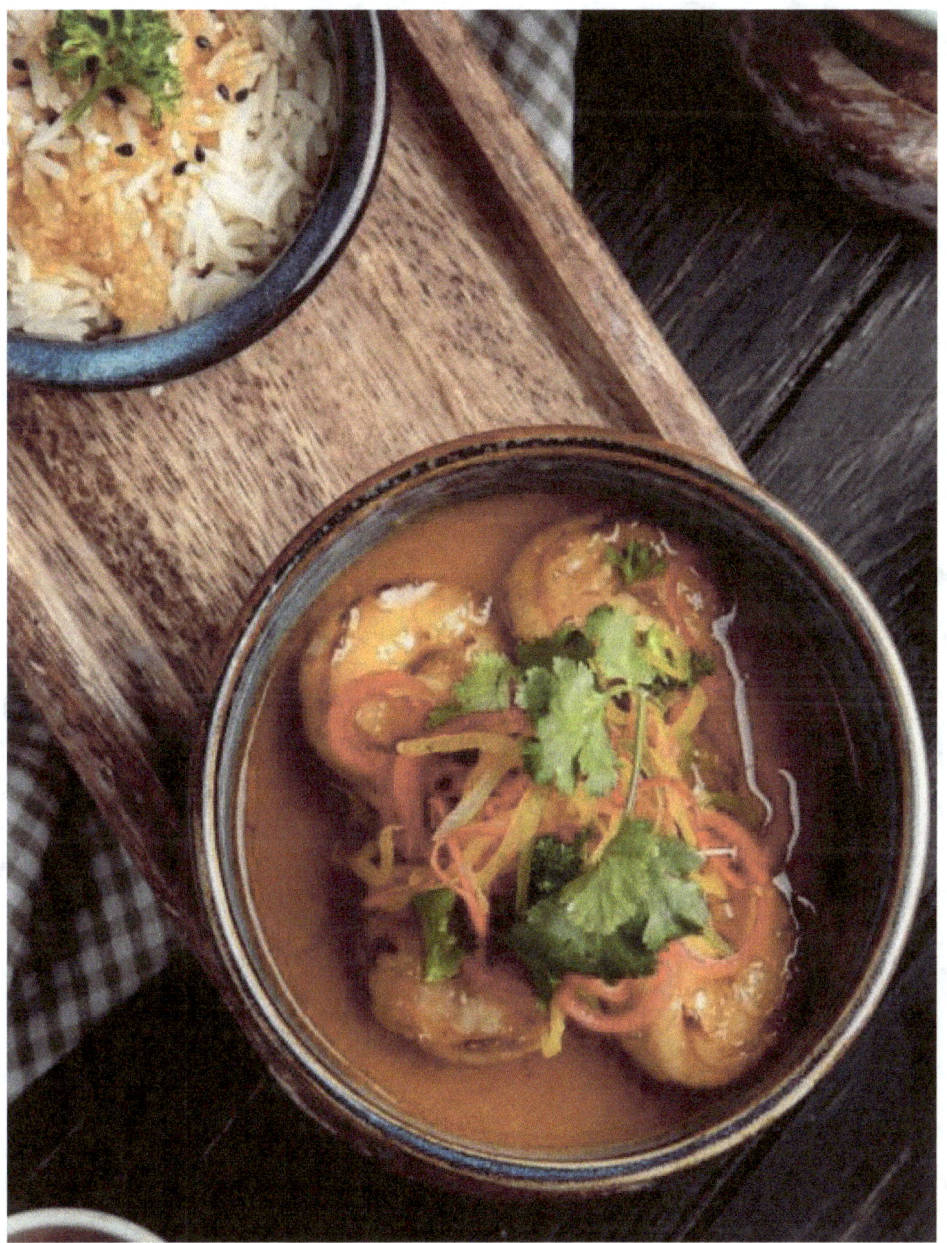

91. Ayam Kicap (Soy Sauce Chicken Stir-Fry)

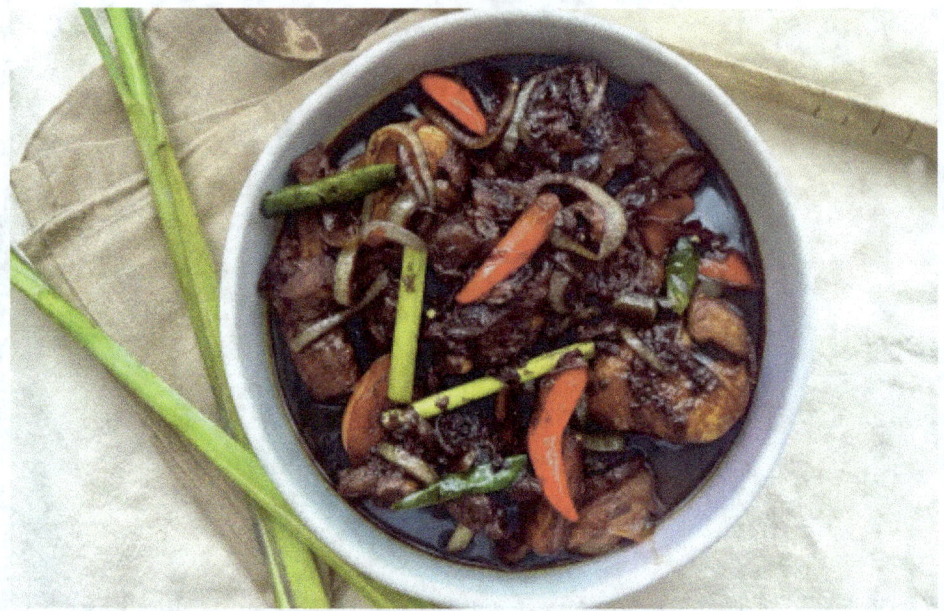

Prep Time: 5 minutes | Cook Time: 10 minutes | Makes: 2

Ayam Kicap is a beloved staple in Malay households, deeply influenced by Chinese and local Malay cooking traditions. Its name simply means "soy sauce chicken," but every family has their own twist on it — from festive braised versions to quick stir-fries. This speedy take delivers the signature sweetness and umami-rich depth using dark soy sauce, garlic, and warm spices, all in under 15 minutes.

INGREDIENTS:
- 200g boneless chicken thighs, thinly sliced
- 2 garlic cloves, minced
- ½ onion, thinly sliced
- 1 tbsp dark soy sauce
- 1 tbsp light soy sauce
- ½ tsp sugar
- ½ tsp chili flakes (optional)
- 1 tbsp oil
- Cooked jasmine rice, to serve

INSTRUCTIONS:
1. Heat oil in a wok. Sauté onions and garlic for 1 minute.
2. Add chicken and cook 5–6 minutes until lightly browned.
3. Stir in dark soy sauce, light soy sauce, sugar, and chili flakes.

4. Simmer 2–3 minutes until sauce thickens slightly.
5. Serve over rice.

NUTRITION ESTIMATES (PER SERVING):
Calories: 460 | Protein: 35g | Carbs: 18g | Fat: 26g | Fiber: 2g

QUICK & EASY TIP: Slice chicken in advance and keep the sauce pre-mixed for quicker execution.

92. Sambal Prawns (Udang Masak Sambal)

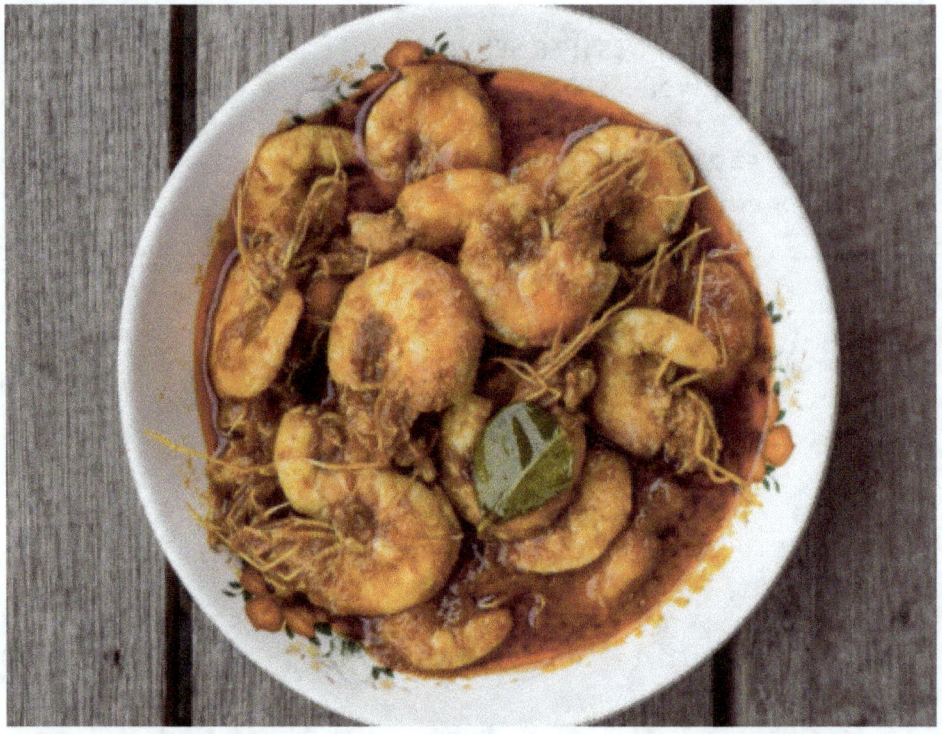

Prep Time: 4 minutes | Cook Time: 10 minutes | Makes: 2

A beloved spicy seafood dish, Sambal Prawns are often served at dinner across Malaysia. It's rich with chili, garlic, and shrimp paste — bold and aromatic. Our shortcut version uses ready-made sambal to reduce cook time dramatically.

INGREDIENTS:
- 200g peeled prawns
- 1½ tbsp sambal oelek (or Malaysian-style sambal)
- 1 garlic clove, minced
- ½ onion, chopped
- ½ tsp sugar
- 1 tbsp oil
- Lime wedges, to serve
- Cooked rice or coconut rice, to serve

INSTRUCTIONS:
1. Heat oil in a pan. Sauté garlic and onion for 2 minutes.
2. Add sambal and sugar. Stir until fragrant.
3. Add prawns and stir-fry 4–5 minutes until cooked through.

4. Serve hot with rice and lime wedges.

NUTRITION ESTIMATES (PER SERVING):
Calories: 410 | Protein: 30g | Carbs: 14g | Fat: 26g | Fiber: 1g

QUICK & EASY TIP: Using pre-peeled prawns and jarred sambal drastically cuts down on prep and cook time.

93. Mee Goreng Mamak (Spicy Fried Noodles)

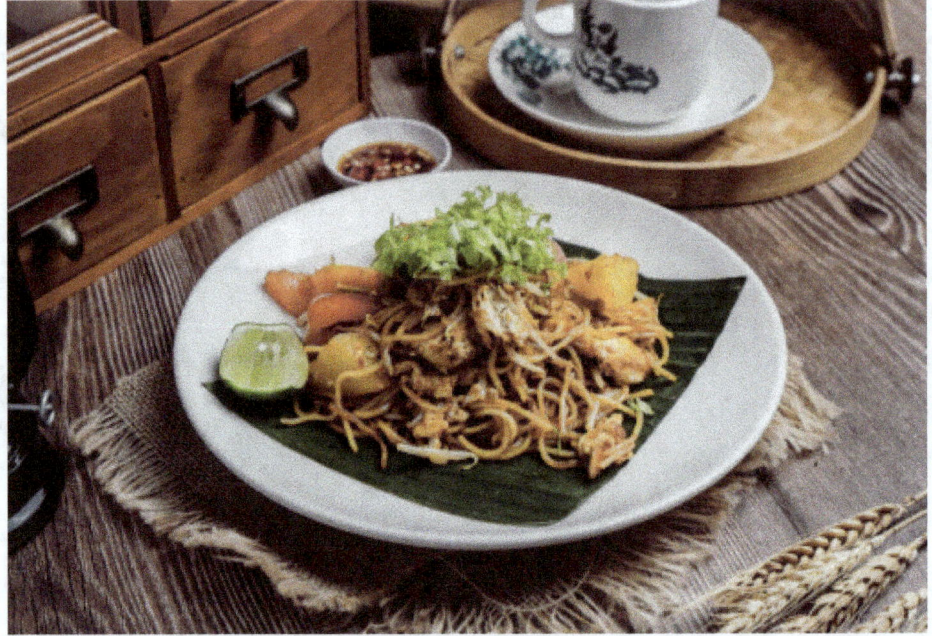

Prep Time: 5 minutes | Cook Time: 9 minutes | Makes: 2

Mee Goreng Mamak is a flavorful noodle stir-fry of Indian-Muslim origin, commonly found at hawker stalls across Malaysia. It blends Chinese-style noodles, Malay ingredients, and Indian spices — the perfect representation of Malaysia's culinary fusion.

INGREDIENTS:
- 200g fresh yellow noodles or cooked instant noodles
- 1 egg
- 100g tofu, cubed
- ½ cup bean sprouts
- 2 garlic cloves, minced
- 1 tbsp soy sauce
- 1 tbsp sweet soy sauce (kecap manis)
- ½ tsp chili paste or sambal
- 1 tbsp oil
- Lime wedges and green onion, to serve

INSTRUCTIONS:
1. Heat oil in a wok. Fry tofu cubes until golden (2–3 mins). Push to side.
2. Crack in the egg, scramble, then add garlic and stir briefly.
3. Add noodles, soy sauces, and chili paste. Stir-fry 2–3 mins.

4. Toss in bean sprouts, stir another 1 minute.
5. Serve with lime and green onion.

NUTRITION ESTIMATES (PER SERVING):
Calories: 520 | Protein: 22g | Carbs: 45g | Fat: 28g | Fiber: 3g

QUICK & EASY TIP: *Use pre-fried tofu or frozen tofu cubes to cut cooking time even more.*

| 94. | Sardine Curry |

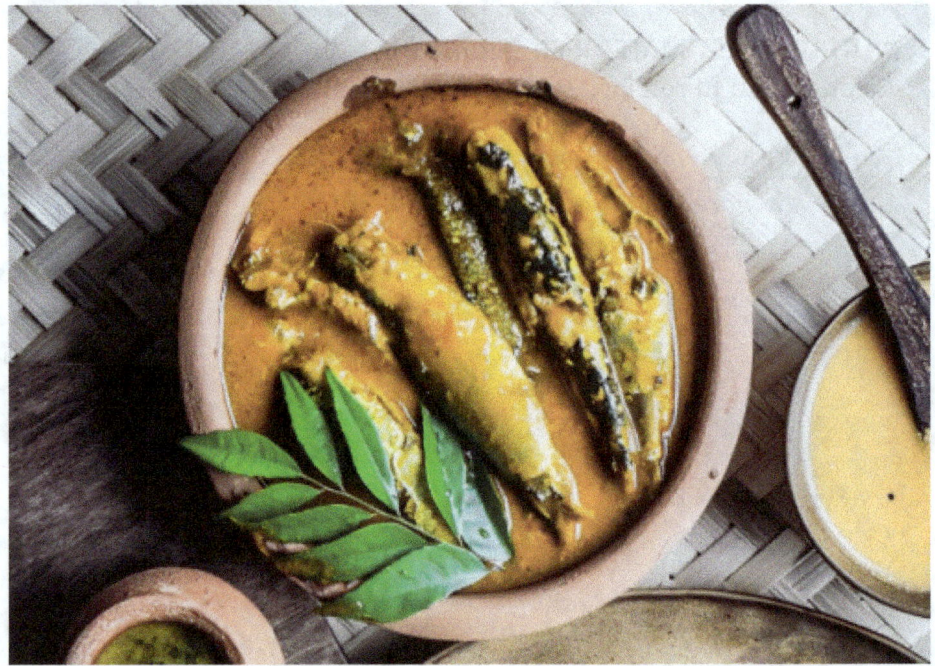

Prep Time: 3 minutes | Cook Time: 10 minutes | Makes: 2

Canned sardine curry, or Kari Sardin Tin, is a true Malaysian classic born out of necessity and ingenuity. Popular among students, busy families, and roadside eateries, it reflects the country's flair for transforming humble pantry staples into deeply flavorful meals. Quick, spicy, and satisfying, this dish showcases how even a simple tin of sardines can become a beloved comfort food.

INGREDIENTS:
- 1 can (155g–200g) sardines in tomato sauce
- ½ onion, sliced
- 1 garlic clove, minced
- 1 tsp curry powder
- ¼ tsp chili powder (optional)
- ½ cup water
- 1 tbsp oil
- Cooked white rice or roti, to serve

INSTRUCTIONS:

1. Heat oil in a pan. Sauté onion and garlic for 2 minutes.
2. Add curry and chili powders. Stir 30 seconds.
3. Add canned sardines with sauce and water.
4. Simmer uncovered for 6–7 minutes until slightly thickened.
5. Serve with rice or roti.

NUTRITION ESTIMATES (PER SERVING):
Calories: 450 | Protein: 28g | Carbs: 16g | Fat: 30g | Fiber: 2g

QUICK & EASY TIP: This is one of the fastest dinners — no chopping if you use pre-sliced onions.

95. Ikan Bakar (Pan-Grilled Fish)

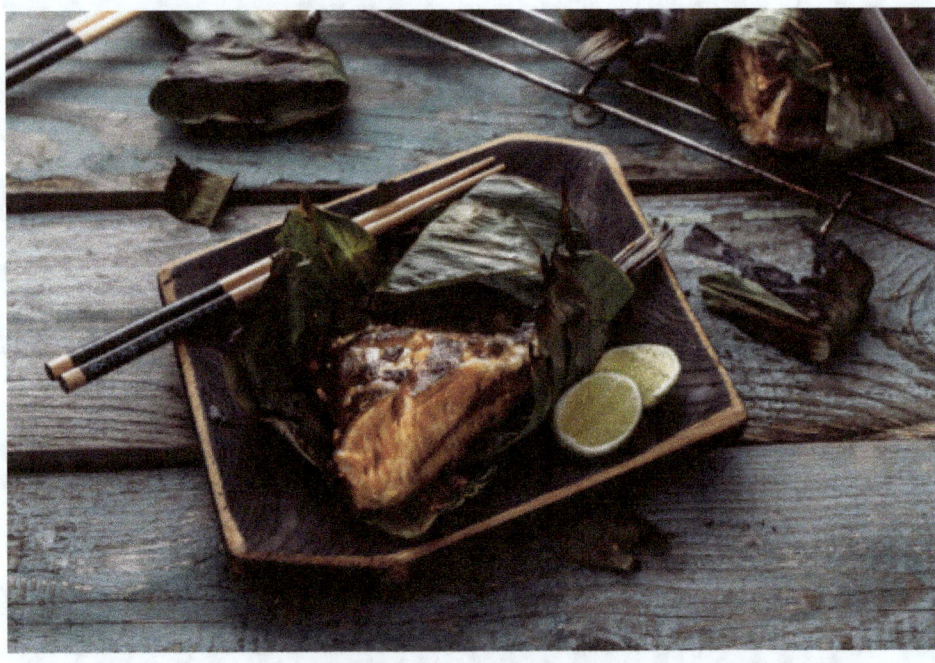

Prep Time: 5 minutes | Cook Time: 9 minutes | Makes: 2

Ikan Bakar, meaning "burnt fish" in Malay, is a cherished street food across Malaysia and Indonesia. Traditionally grilled over open flames and wrapped in banana leaves, the fish absorbs smoky aromas and spicy-sweet sambal flavors. This quick pan-seared version brings the essence of night market grilling into your kitchen — no charcoal required. Just add a squeeze of lime and you're instantly transported to Southeast Asia.

INGREDIENTS:
- 2 small fish fillets (e.g., tilapia, snapper)
- 2 tbsp sambal or chili paste
- 1 tsp lime juice
- ½ tsp sugar
- 1 tbsp oil
- Salt, to taste
- Lime wedges and rice, to serve

INSTRUCTIONS:
1. Mix sambal, lime juice, and sugar. Rub mixture over fish.
2. Heat oil in a non-stick pan. Sear fish for 3–4 minutes per side until cooked through.
3. Serve with lime wedges and hot rice.

NUTRITION ESTIMATES (PER SERVING):
Calories: 390 | Protein: 30g | Carbs: 10g | Fat: 25g | Fiber: 1g

QUICK & EASY TIP: Use boneless fillets and store-bought sambal for ultra-fast prep and cleanup.

96. Malaysian Chicken Kurma

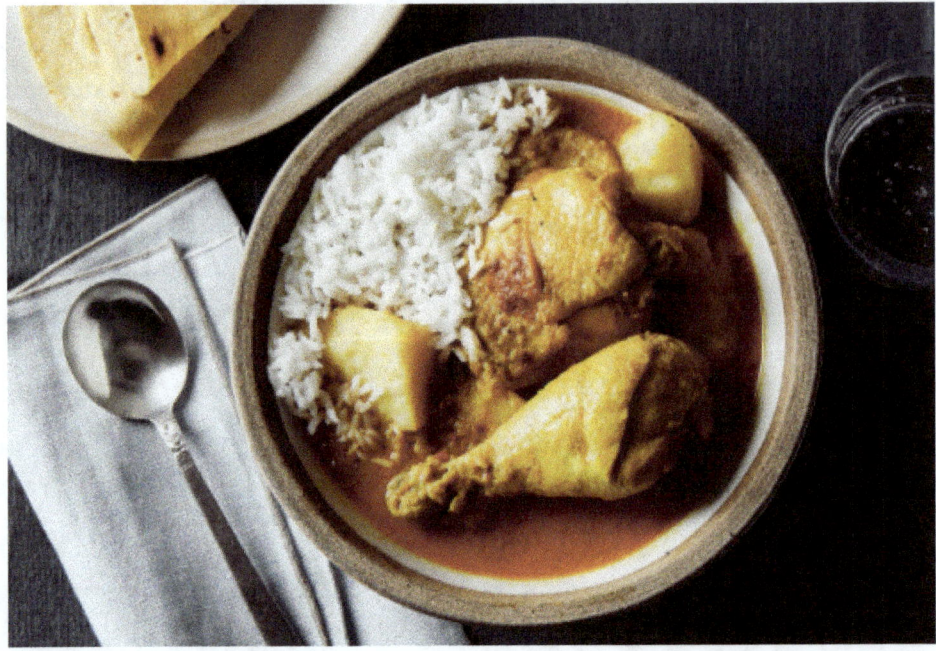

Prep Time: 4 minutes | Cook Time: 10 minutes | Makes: 2

Kurma Ayam is a beloved dish from Malaysia's diverse culinary heritage, influenced by Indian Mughlai cuisine and adapted over centuries by Malay cooks. Unlike the fiery curries of the region, this version is milder—creamy, fragrant, and often prepared for weddings, Eid, and family celebrations. Traditionally slow-cooked with whole spices, this quick adaptation uses boneless chicken and coconut milk for full flavor in a fraction of the time.

INGREDIENTS:
- 200g boneless chicken, diced
- ¼ onion, finely chopped
- 1 garlic clove, minced
- 1 tsp ginger paste
- 1 tsp kurma or mild curry powder
- 100ml coconut milk
- 1 tbsp oil
- Salt, to taste
- Cooked rice or paratha, to serve

INSTRUCTIONS:

1. Heat oil in a pan. Sauté onion, garlic, and ginger paste for 1–2 minutes.
2. Add chicken and kurma powder. Stir and cook for 5–6 minutes.
3. Pour in coconut milk. Simmer 2–3 minutes until thickened.
4. Serve with rice or flatbread.

NUTRITION ESTIMATES (PER SERVING):
Calories: 470 | Protein: 32g | Carbs: 12g | Fat: 32g | Fiber: 1g

<u>*QUICK & EASY TIP:*</u> *Buy pre-cut chicken and ready-mixed kurma spice for a true time-saver dinner.*

KOREAN DINNERS

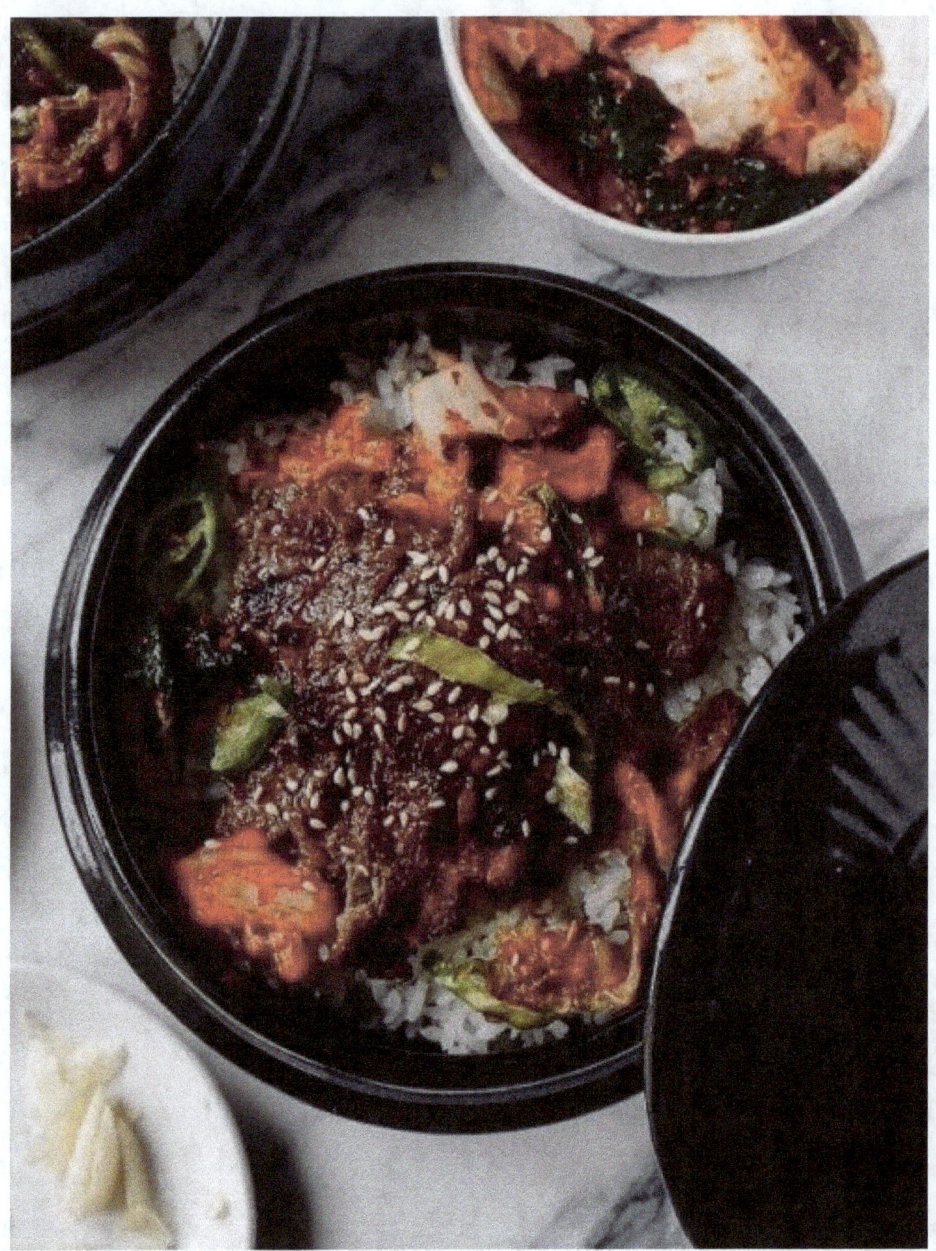

97. Bulgogi Beef Skillet

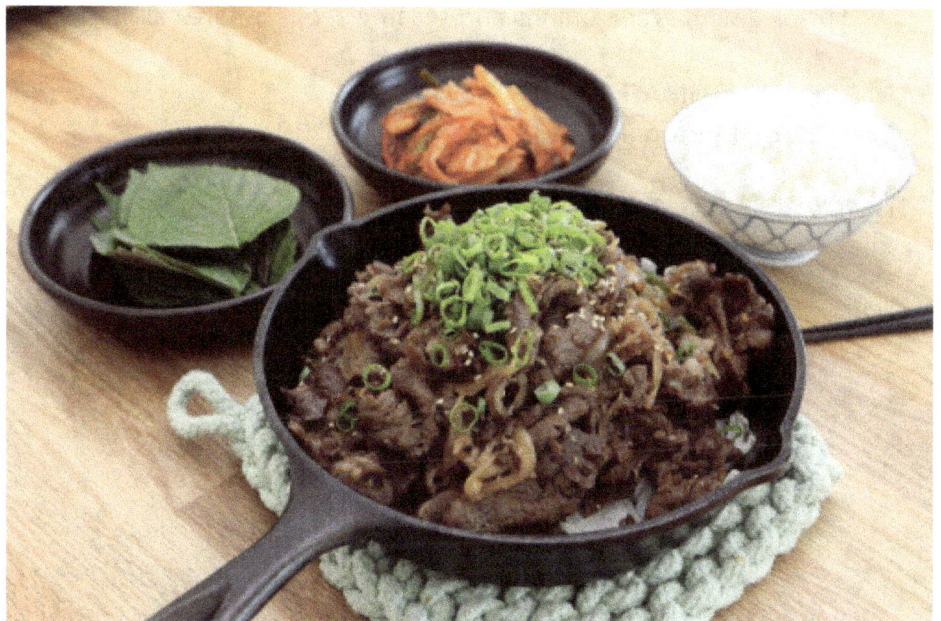

Prep Time: 7 minutes | Cook Time: 7 minutes | Makes: 2

A classic Korean dish meaning "fire meat," Bulgogi is thinly sliced beef marinated in a sweet-savory blend of soy sauce, garlic, sesame oil, and sugar. Traditionally grilled, this quick stir-fried version brings all the flavor in less time, making it a beloved weeknight dinner across Korean households.

INGREDIENTS:
- 200g beef sirloin, thinly sliced
- 2 tbsp soy sauce
- 1 tbsp brown sugar
- 1 tbsp sesame oil
- 2 garlic cloves, minced
- 1/2 small onion, sliced
- 1 green onion, sliced
- 1/2 tsp grated ginger
- 1/2 tsp sesame seeds
- 1 tsp vegetable oil

INSTRUCTIONS:
1. In a bowl, mix soy sauce, brown sugar, sesame oil, garlic, and ginger.
2. Add sliced beef and onions. Marinate for at least 5 minutes.

3. Heat vegetable oil in a skillet over high heat.
4. Add beef mixture and stir-fry for 4–5 minutes until cooked through.
5. Sprinkle with green onions and sesame seeds before serving.

NUTRITION ESTIMATES (PER SERVING):
Calories: 320 | Protein: 28g | Carbs: 10g | Fat: 19g

<u>**QUICK & EASY TIP:**</u> *Use pre-sliced beef or ask your butcher to do it—huge time saver.*

98. Kimchi Fried Rice (Kimchi Bokkeumbap)

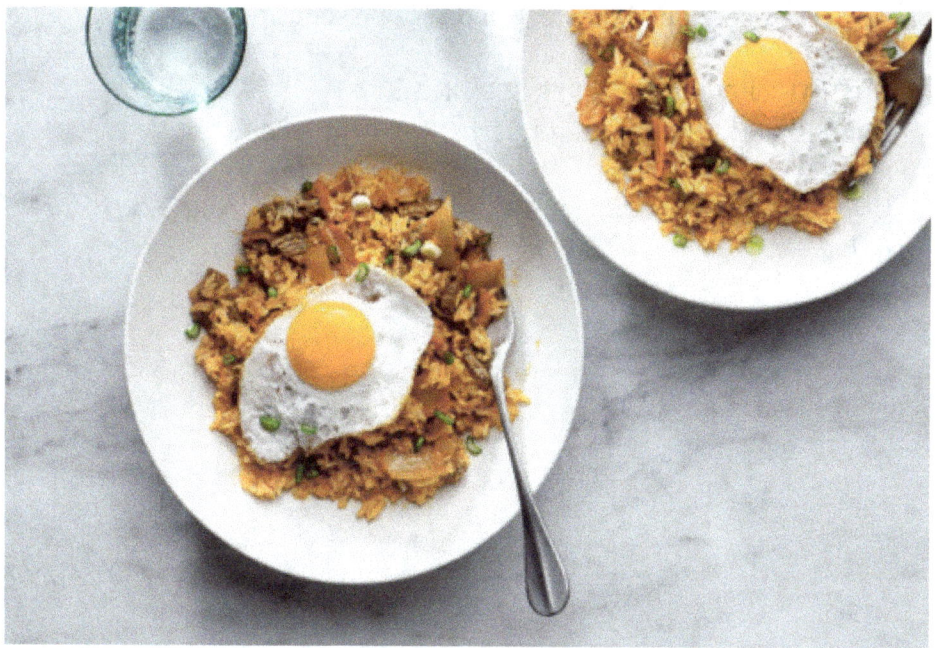

Prep Time: 5 minutes | Cook Time: 10 minutes | Makes: 2

This spicy, tangy fried rice is a genius way to use leftover rice and kimchi. A pantry staple in Korea, it's ready in minutes and often topped with a fried egg for a satisfying, umami-rich dinner.

INGREDIENTS:
- 1 cup kimchi, chopped
- 1 tbsp kimchi juice (from the jar)
- 2 cups cold cooked rice
- 1 tbsp gochujang (Korean chili paste)
- 1 tbsp soy sauce
- 2 green onions, chopped
- 1 tbsp vegetable oil
- 1 tsp sesame oil
- 2 eggs (optional)
- Sesame seeds (for garnish)

INSTRUCTIONS:
1. Heat vegetable oil in a skillet over medium-high heat.
2. Sauté kimchi for 2–3 minutes. Add kimchi juice, gochujang, and soy sauce.
3. Add rice and stir-fry for 5 minutes until well combined.

4. Stir in green onions and sesame oil.
5. In a separate pan, fry eggs sunny-side up (if using).
6. Serve rice topped with egg and sesame seeds.

NUTRITION ESTIMATES (PER SERVING):
Calories: 390 | Protein: 12g | Carbs: 42g | Fat: 18g

QUICK & EASY TIP: *Cold leftover rice prevents clumping—perfect for fast frying.*

99. Gochujang Chicken Stir-Fry

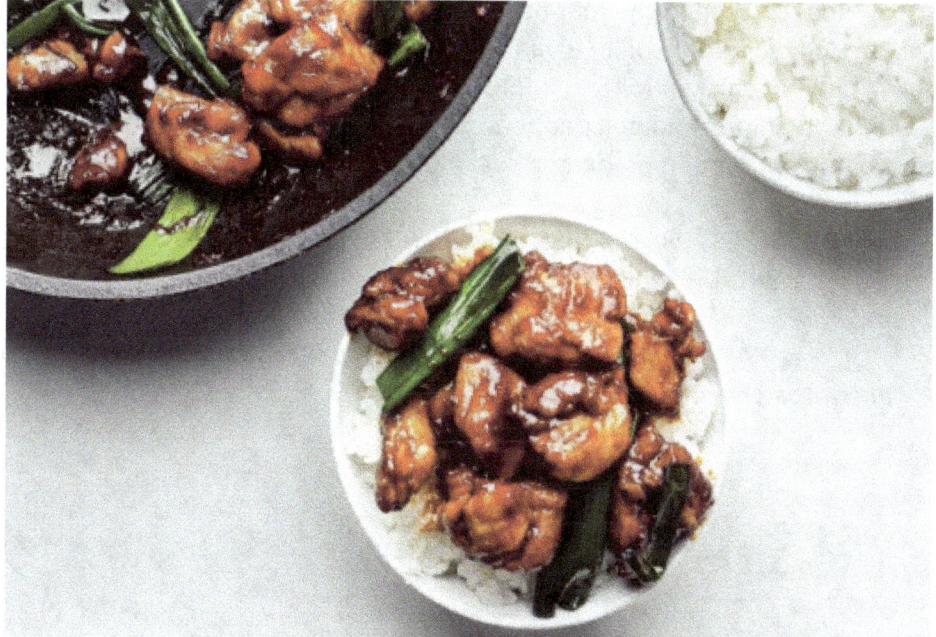

Prep Time: 5 minutes | Cook Time: 10 minutes | Makes: 2

Gochujang, Korea's iconic red chili paste, dates back to the 16th century when chili peppers were first introduced to the region. Traditionally fermented for months in clay pots, this spicy-sweet condiment brings deep umami and heat to countless Korean dishes. In this fast stir-fry, gochujang stars as the bold sauce that coats tender chicken, making it a quick nod to Korea's vibrant street food scene — best enjoyed with rice or lettuce wraps.

INGREDIENTS:
- 250g boneless chicken thighs, thinly sliced
- 1 tbsp gochujang (Korean chili paste)
- 1 tbsp soy sauce
- 1 tsp honey or sugar
- 2 garlic cloves, minced
- 1 tsp sesame oil
- 1 tbsp vegetable oil
- 1/2 onion, sliced
- 1/2 bell pepper, sliced
- 1 green onion, chopped
- Sesame seeds, for garnish

INSTRUCTIONS:
1. In a bowl, mix gochujang, soy sauce, honey, garlic, and sesame oil.
2. Toss chicken in the marinade and let sit while prepping vegetables.
3. Heat vegetable oil in a pan over medium-high heat.
4. Stir-fry chicken for 5–6 minutes until cooked through.
5. Add onions and bell peppers. Cook for another 2–3 minutes.
6. Top with green onion and sesame seeds. Serve hot.

NUTRITION ESTIMATES (PER SERVING):
Calories: 340 | Protein: 29g | Carbs: 10g | Fat: 21g

<u>*QUICK & EASY TIP:*</u> *Using pre-cut chicken speeds up prep. You can also batch the sauce for future use.*

100.   Korean Tofu Stew (Sundubu Jjigae)

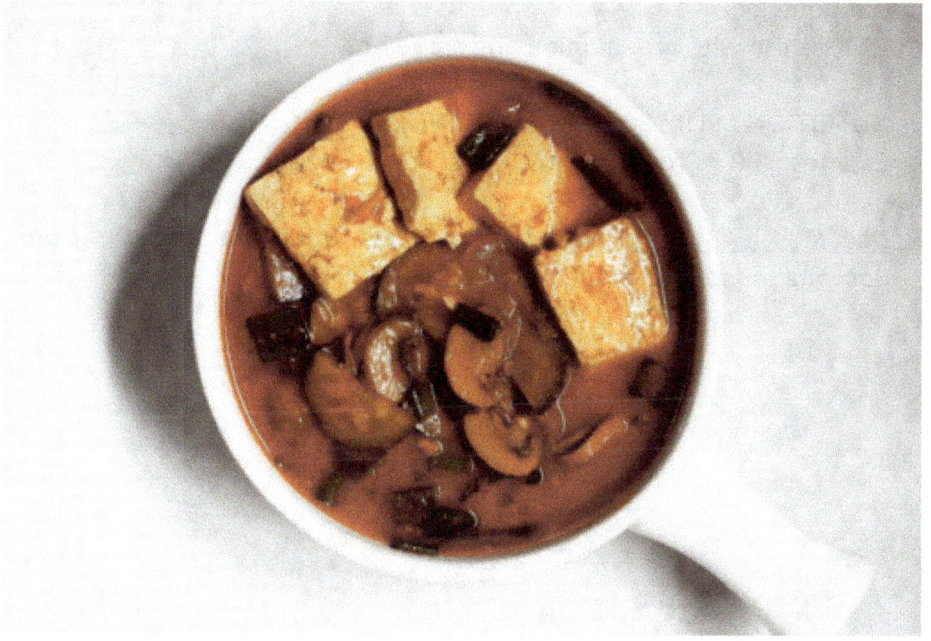

Prep Time: 5 minutes | Cook Time: 10 minutes | Makes: 2

A streamlined version of Korea's comforting soft tofu stew. Made without seafood or slow-cooked broth, this quick version keeps all the warmth and depth in a fraction of the time.

INGREDIENTS:
- 200g silken tofu (soft tofu)
- 1/2 small onion, diced
- 1 green onion, chopped
- 2 garlic cloves, minced
- 1 tsp gochugaru (Korean red pepper flakes)
- 1 tbsp soy sauce
- 1/2 tsp sesame oil
- 1 tbsp vegetable oil
- 1/2 cup vegetable or chicken broth
- 1 egg (optional)

INSTRUCTIONS:
1. Heat vegetable oil in a small pot. Add onions and garlic. Sauté for 2–3 minutes.
2. Add gochugaru, soy sauce, sesame oil, and stir.
3. Pour in broth and bring to a simmer.

4. Gently add silken tofu in large chunks.
5. Let simmer 5 minutes. Add egg on top and cook for 1–2 minutes (optional).
6. Garnish with green onion and serve hot.

NUTRITION ESTIMATES (PER SERVING):
Calories: 260 | Protein: 14g | Carbs: 7g | Fat: 20g

QUICK & EASY TIP: *No need to press tofu—use straight from the package for speed.*

CONCLUSION

Thank you for inviting this cookbook into your kitchen and trusting it to guide your evenings. Whether you've flipped through these pages out of necessity, curiosity, or a craving for something new, we're so glad you came along for the journey.

What you now hold isn't just a collection of 15-minute recipes — it's a celebration of global traditions, time-saving wisdom, and the simple magic of a home-cooked meal. From Thai stir-fries and Italian skillet pastas to Middle Eastern classics and Latin-inspired wraps, you've just cooked your way around the world in under 15 minutes at a time.

More than that, you've embraced a new way to think about dinner: one that's flexible, flavorful, and never intimidating. You've discovered that real food doesn't have to take hours, that one pan can be enough, and that cultural exploration can begin at your stovetop. Along the way, you've learned shortcuts, mastered quick-prep ingredients, and stocked a kitchen that works for your life — not against it.

Let this cookbook be more than a one-time flip-through. Come back to it on busy weeknights, low-energy days, or when you just need a little inspiration. Let it remind you that dinner doesn't have to be complicated to be memorable — and that the act of cooking, even quickly, can still feel deeply grounding.

So here's to your next 15-minute dinner. May it be delicious, stress-free, and shared with someone you love — even if that someone is just you, standing over the stove with a fork in one hand and satisfaction in the other.

Bon appétit. And once again — thank you.